Clinical Diagnosis and Management of Squamous Cell Carcinoma

Edited by Sivapatham Sundaresan

Published in London, United Kingdom

Clinical Diagnosis and Management of Squamous Cell Carcinoma
http://dx.doi.org/10.5772/intechopen.94812
Edited by Sivapatham Sundaresan

Contributors
Sahana Ashok, Chanyoot Bandidwattanawong, Chau-Yin Chen, Jin-Jhe Wang, Yueh-Ju Tsai, Sivasamy Ramasamy, Minu Jenifer Michael Raj, Fenwick Antony Edwin Rodrigues, Ferhat Cetin, Özer Birge, Runjhun Mathur, Niraj Kumar Jha, Saurabh Kumar Jha, Mehak Sharan, Khushboo Rana, Abhimanyu Kumar Jha, Sivapatham Sundaresan, Lavanya Selvaraj

First published in London, United Kingdom, 2023 by IntechOpen
IntechOpen is the global imprint of INTECHOPEN LIMITED, registered in England and Wales, registration number: 11086078, 5 Princes Gate Court, London, SW7 2QJ, United Kingdom

British Library Cataloguing-in-Publication Data
A catalogue record for this book is available from the British Library

Additional hard and PDF copies can be obtained from orders@intechopen.com

Clinical Diagnosis and Management of Squamous Cell Carcinoma
Edited by Sivapatham Sundaresan
p. cm.
Print ISBN 978-1-80355-540-9
Online ISBN 978-1-80355-541-6
eBook (PDF) ISBN 978-1-80355-542-3

Meet the editor

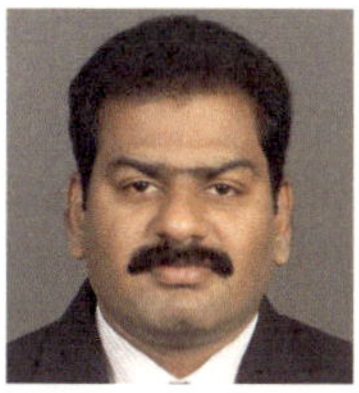

Dr. Sivapatham Sundaresan is an associate professor in the Department of Medical Research at the SRM Medical College Hospital and Research Center and SRM Institute of Science and Technology, India. He works on cancer chemoprevention, cancer immunotherapy and tumor marker detection. Recent research interest is the impact of probiotics on the treatment of intestinal toxicity during chemotherapy and its adjunct role in colorectal cancer. He is a member of the Indian Association of Clinical Biochemists and has published many papers in national and international journals.

Contents

Preface

Squamous cell carcinomas (SCC) are a group of cancers that originate from cells within the epidermis. SCC is the cause of about 90% of cases of head and neck cancer, which includes cancers of the mouth, nasal cavity, nasopharynx, throat, and related non-small cell lung cancer. This book reviews squamous cell carcinoma of the bladder, eye, vagina, and head and neck, examines the site-specific importance of the disease and discusses the application of dermatoscopy and the role of Next Generation Sequencing in SCC. The mutational profile of human papillomavirus (HPV) in head and neck SCC as a source for cancer diagnosis and management is discussed. Numerous studies have shown that the consumption of raw fruits and vegetables significantly reduces the risk of SCC, and green leafy vegetables may aid in the prevention of SCC development.

Sivapatham Sundaresan
Associate Professor,
SRM Institute of Science and Technology,
Chennai, India

Chapter 1

Squamous Cell Carcinoma of the Vagina

Ferhat Cetin and Özer Birge

Abstract

Vaginal cancer accounts for approximately 4000 cases and over 900 deaths annually. About 1 in 100,000 women will be diagnosed with in situ or invasive vaginal cancer (typically of squamous cell histology). The mean age at diagnosis of squamous cell carcinoma, the most common histologic type of vaginal cancer, is approximately 60 years. However, the disease is seen occasionally in women in their 20s and 30s. Squamous carcinoma is more common as the age of the patient increases. Vaginal cancer is a disease in which malignant (cancer) cells form in the vagina. Vaginal cancer is staged in three ways, based on how far the tumor has progressed in the vagina, whether it has spread to the lymph nodes, and whether it has spread to other parts of the body. These three categories are called T (tumor), N (nodes), and M (whether it has metastasized or spread). Surgery is the most common treatment of vaginal cancer. The surgical procedures used are laser surgery (uses a laser beam as a knife to make bloodless cuts in tissue or to remove a surface lesion such as a tumor); Wide local excision (takes out cancer and some of the healthy tissue around it); Vaginectomy (Surgery to remove all or part of the vagina).

Keywords: human papillomavirus, primary vaginal cancer, squamous cell carcinoma, vaginal bleeding

1. Introduction

Primary vaginal cancer is less prevalent than uterine cancer of the endometrium, ovary, and cervix, but vaginal cancer is more common than vulvar cancer in the United States [1]. Most vaginal tumors are squamous cell carcinomas, but melanomas, sarcomas, adenocarcinomas, and other histologic types also occur. Although primary vaginal cancer is rare, metastasis to the vagina or local spread from adjacent gynecologic or non-gynecologic organs or systems is not uncommon.

In summary, most vaginal malignancies are metastatic and can often arise from the endometrium, cervix, vulva, ovaries, breast, rectum, and kidney [2–5]. Direct spread (e.g., cervix, vulva, endometrium) or lymphatic or hematogenous spread (e.g., breast, ovary, kidney) can cause vaginal metastases.

In situ or invasive vaginal cancer will be diagnosed in approximately one in every 100,000 women (typically squamous cell histology) [6, 7]. Squamous cell carcinoma, the most frequent histologic form of vaginal cancer, is mainly diagnosed in women in their 60s and 70s, while it can also occur in women in their 20s and 30s. Squamous cell carcinoma occurs more frequently as the patient ages [6].

Human papillomavirus (HPV) infection is thought to be the cause of the majority of vaginal cancer cases, as well as cervical, uterine cancer [8]. In a case–control study, more than half of 156 women with in situ or invasive vaginal cancer tested positive for antibodies to HPV 16 or 18 subtypes [9]. As a result, vaginal cancer and cervical neoplasia share the same risk factors. Specifically, the risk increases with more than one sexual partner over a lifetime, early age at first sexual intercourse, if you still smoke, low socioeconomic status, and various other infections that cause immunosuppression [9, 10].

There was evidence that some high-grade vulvar and vaginal intraepithelial neoplasms are monoclonal lesions derived from the high-grade or malignant disease of the cervix [11]. A retrospective cohort study of over 130,000 women found that women with cervical intraepithelial neoplasia 3 (CIN 3) had a significantly higher risk of developing vaginal cancer than women in the same population and time interval (incidence rate 6.8, 95% CI 5.6–8.2) [12]. A fourfold or higher risk was found up to 25 years after a CIN 3 diagnosis. Similarly, 30% of all women with in situ or invasive vaginal disease had previously been treated for an anogenital tumor (primarily cervical), and 17 out of 25 (70%) invasive cancer biopsy specimens tested positive for HPV type 16/18 DNA in one case series. Similarly, 51 of 153 women with vaginal cancer treated at Princess Margaret Hospital had pre-existing gynecological malignancies, 34 of whom had cervical uteri cancer, and it is recommended that when each type of cancer is detected, the cervix uteri, vagina, and vulvar region be evaluated together [13].

2. Clinical findings

The most prevalent clinical manifestation of vaginal cancer is vaginal bleeding. Many women are asymptomatic. Vaginal bleeding associated with vaginal cancer is typically postcoital or postmenopausal. Any unplanned vaginal bleeding should be investigated to determine if the source is vaginal. There may also be a watery, bloody, or foul-smelling discharge from the vagina [14–16].

The patient may also notice a vaginal mass. Other possible symptoms are related to local spread of the disease, urinary symptoms (e.g., frequency, dysuria, hematuria), or gastrointestinal symptoms (e.g., tenesmus, constipation, melena) [14–16]. Pelvic pain caused by the spread of the disease outside the vagina occurs in 5 percent of patients.

At the time of diagnosis, up to 20% of women have no clinical complaints and are asymptomatic [17–19]. These vaginal malignancies might be discovered incidentally during a pelvic examination or due to cytological screening for cervical cancer.

3. Diagnostic evaluation

Evaluation using pelvic examination, vaginal cytology, and colposcopic or direct vaginal biopsy are the essential parts of diagnostic evaluation.

Questions about the symptoms of vaginal cancer should be included. A gynecologic history, including a history of neoplasms of the cervix or vulvar neoplasia, should be obtained, as a history of other gynecologic malignancies may exclude a diagnosis of vaginal cancer. Medical, surgical, and medication history should be obtained. This should include the evaluation of medical comorbidities that may influence treatment decisions.

A pelvic and physical examination is carried out. The vagina should be extensively checked with the speculum, including the view of the entire periphery and fornix by shifting the speculum position. Any abnormal site or mass should be biopsied. Palpation of the vaginal walls for masses and evaluation of other pelvic masses should be included in a bimanual examination. The inguinal region should be palpated to assess enlarged pathological lymph nodes.

If the lesion is small and located in the lower two-thirds of the vagina, it may be missed on initial examination. On visual inspection of the vagina, the anterior and posterior blades of the speculum obscure this area, so the tumor may be missed unless the vagina is examined when the speculum is removed or the lesion is palpated on bimanual examination. A detailed colposcopic examination is recommended for macroscopic lesions or lesions that cannot be seen with the naked eye.

The rectovaginal examination is also recommended to assess parametrial and pelvic sidewall involvement, as well as probable rectal involvement.

The most prevalent site of primary vaginal carcinoma is the posterior wall of the upper third of the vagina. According to review research, more than half of the tumors in the upper, middle, and lower thirds of the vaginal wall originated in the posterior vaginal wall in 50, 20, and 30% of cases, respectively [7, 20]. A mass, plaque, or ulcer can all be signs of a lesion. To assess metastatic disease, a focused physical examination is conducted. The inguinal region, in particular, should be checked for pathologically enlarged lymph nodes.

A vaginal cytology specimen should be obtained during the pelvic examination. Twenty percent of vaginal cancers are discovered incidentally during cytology screening for cervical cancer [21].

If a lesion cannot be visualized and cytology results are abnormal, acetic acid colposcopy of the cervix and vagina should be performed, followed by Lugol's iodine staining. If a large lesion is visible, some specialists additionally recommend vaginal colposcopy to evaluate the rest of the vagina.

Biopsy of abnormal areas of the vagina in the office may be performed with punch forceps (Baker or Keyes) or cervical biopsy forceps (Tischler or Burke). Examination under anesthesia may be required for examination and biopsy in women with the significant vaginal stricture that prevents adequate office examination, older adult women, or if cystoscopy and proctoscopy are required for clinical staging.

The only imaging studies part of the International Federation of Gynecology and Obstetrics (FIGO) staging for vaginal cancer are chest and skeletal radiographs.

Modern imaging techniques, such as computed tomography (CT), magnetic resonance imaging (MRI), and 18-fluoro-2-deoxyglucose-positron emission tomography and CT (FDG-PET/CT), can help plan treatment. MRI may help determine the size and local extent of the primary vaginal tumor [22, 23]. T2 imaging is usually the best way to see vaginal tumors, and dripping gel into the vaginal canal to expand the vaginal walls can help visualize and evaluate the tumor's thickness. Primary vaginal tumors and abnormal lymph nodes can also be assessed using FDG-PET [24].

4. Diagnosis

Vaginal cancer is a histologic diagnosis based on vaginal biopsy and the absence of a history of gynecologic malignancy may better identify the vaginal disease as recurrent cancer rather than a new primary disease.

4.1 Differential diagnosis

The first step in determining the cause of vaginal bleeding is to rule out bleeding from other areas of the genital tract. A pelvic examination is often used to accomplish this.

Menopausal women may experience vaginal bleeding due to vaginal atrophy. Bleeding can also be caused by a vaginal infection, inflammation, or trauma. A dermatological condition occasionally causes vaginal bleeding (e.g., toxic epidermal necrolysis). Bleeding from these etiologies may result in focal bleeding from a fissure or laceration, which is not usually the case with vaginal cancer. Or there may be ulceration or extensive bleeding, which can also occur with vaginal cancer. A vaginal mass may be benign, such as cysts of the ductus Gartner, vaginal polyps, vaginal adenosis, endometriosis, or dermoid cysts (rare) [25].

4.2 Histopathology

Primary vaginal tumors form a heterogeneous group of malignancies. They may be multicentric and involve many areas, so the entire vaginal mucosa is at risk and should be examined.

The majority of vaginal cancers are squamous cell carcinomas. As previously stated, the average age at diagnosis for squamous cell carcinomas is around 60 years [26]. Tumors can be nodular, ulcerative, indurated, endophytic, or exophytic in general. They resemble squamous cell tumors in other regions histologically. Vaginal cancer is also associated with the human papillomavirus (HPV). The vaginal epithelium, on the other hand, is more stable than the cervical epithelium, which undergoes constant metaplasia and is hence less susceptible to oncogenic viruses [27].

Verrucous carcinoma is an uncommon type of vaginal squamous cell carcinoma that is well-differentiated and has a small probability of becoming malignant [28]. It is usually a large, warty, fungal mass that is locally aggressive but rarely metastasizes. Histologically, it consists of large papillary sheets covered with dense keratin. The deep margin forms a driving edge of well-aligned rete ridges, in contrast to the well-demarcated margins of benign condyloma acuminata.

4.3 Staging

A clinical staging system for vaginal cancer is used by the International Federation of Gynecology and Obstetrics (FIGO) and Tumor, Node, and Metastasis (TNM) [29–31].

Physical examination, cystoscopy, proctoscopy, and chest and skeletal radiographs are used to determine clinical staging. The results of biopsy or fine-needle aspiration of inguinal/femoral nodes or other nodules may be included in the clinical stage. In addition to clinical staging data, information from the resected specimen, including pelvic and peritoneal lymph nodes, will be used as indicated by the TNM system.

In a review of five series with 1375 cases of vaginal cancer, patients were differentiated according to FIGO stage: stage I (26%), stage II (37%), stage III (24%), and stage IV (13%) [32].

Vaginal tumors can spread locally and in various ways systemically:

- Direct extension to the soft tissue structures of the pelvis: parameters, bladder, urethra, and rectum. Eventually, the bony pelvis may also be affected.

- Lymphatic spread to the pelvic and para-aortic lymph nodes. The lymphatic drainage of the upper vagina connects with the cervix and continues first to the pelvic nodes and then to the paraaortic nodes. In comparison, the lymphatics of the distal third of the vagina drain first to the inguinal and femoral nodes and secondarily to the pelvic nodes.

- Hematogenous spread to other organs, including lungs, liver, and bone, is usually seen late and in histopathologically rare lesions.

4.4 Treatment

Because of its rarity, no randomized trials describe the treatment of vaginal cancer. Instead, the treatment approach of cervical and anal cancer is predicted. In addition, treatment plans should be individualized according to the tumor's location, size, and clinical stage. This was supported by a review from a single institution, which showed that tumor stage, location, and size were significant prognostic factors in patients with vaginal cancer [33]. In addition, treatment should consider the following:

- Local anatomic constraints (e.g., removal of internal genitalia, supporting structures, rectosigmoid, lymphatics, and bladder) prevent wide negative surgical margins without an exenterative surgery.

- Psychosexual problems, including the patient's desire to obtain a functioning vagina.

- For most patients with **stage I tumors**, we recommend surgical excision. However, radiation therapy (RT) may be appropriate in some patients, especially for tumors >2 cm or lesions involving the mid to lower vagina.

- Radiotherapy is also used for tumors in the mid to lower vagina because of anatomic difficulties, as surgical resection of tumors at this site often requires vulvovaginectomy and inguinal node dissection to achieve negative margins and acceptable oncologic outcomes [34]. On the other hand, surgical resection is more appropriate for patients with lesions in the upper posterior vagina because the anatomy is preserved.

- We usually prefer RT to surgery because negative margins are difficult to achieve in tumors bigger than 2 to 3 cm in diameter [35]. Even if surgical resection is performed, obtaining an appropriate margin is challenging if the lesion is located close to the bladder or rectum.

If the tumor is located in the distal part of the vagina, the inguinal lymph nodes should also be examined.

Surgical: A radical hysterectomy, upper vaginectomy, and bilateral pelvic lymphadenectomy are required for the vaginal cancer approach. If hysterectomy has been performed previously, radical vaginectomy and bilateral lymphadenectomy should be performed to complete surgical treatment. When patients with stage I vaginal cancer are treated surgically, they appear to have the best results. This was supported by a literature review that showed that patients with early-stage disease had a median five-year survival rate of 77%, much better than that of patients with late-stage disease, whether or not adjuvant RT was applied [6, 36].

Radiation therapy: For some patients, radiation alone is a sufficient treatment. For example, in a series of 91 women treated at a single institution, results obtained with modern RT for early-stage vaginal cancer were shown: In stage I patients (n = 38), the two-year overall survival rate, regional control rate, and distant metastasis-free survival rate were 96.2%, 80.6%, and 87.5%, respectively [20]. More than 2500 vaginal cancer patients were studied in the Surveillance, Epidemiology, and End Results (SEER) trial, which indicated that treatment with brachytherapy was better with 3.6 median survival years, rather than 6.1 years with external radiation alone [37].

A total radiation dose of at least 70 to 75 Gy is commonly suggested, with 45 to 50 Gy of external beam radiation and additional radiation provided via intracavitary or interstitial brachytherapy radiation, depending on the thickness of the primary tumor. Pelvic lymph nodes rimmed vaginal tumors, vaginal and paravaginal tissues, and inguinal lymph nodes should all be exposed to external radiation if the vaginal tumor is in the lower half of the vaginal canal. Brachytherapy radiation should be given immediately after the completion of external radiation. Vaginal tumors less than 5 mm thick can be treated using a vaginal roller or similar applicator, however tumors thicker than 5 mm require interstitial therapy for appropriate dosage and normal tissue preservation [38].

Surgery is usually not an option for patients with more advanced stages than II to IV. We frequently replace chemoradiotherapy for RT because of the relatively poor results of RT alone. However, given the lack of high-quality data on the benefits of chemoradiation, RT is a reasonable alternative, especially for patients who, for some reason, are not eligible for cisplatin-based chemotherapy.

Chemoradiation: In patients with advanced vaginal cancer, concurrent use of RT with chemotherapy (fluorouracil [FU] and/or cisplatin) is our preferred approach due to the usual issues associated with central tumor control. Because of the poor prognosis with radiation alone (predominantly local failures) [39], we often proceed to the combined use of radiation and concomitant chemotherapy in women with high-risk disease (e.g., stage III or IV or tumor size greater than 4) [40–42]. This is mainly based on extrapolating better results with chemoradiation for locally advanced cervical cancer treatment.

There are few data to support this approach, particularly in vaginal cancer, and these are mostly limited to small retrospective series [40, 42–44], which consistently show high rates of locoregional control after chemoradiotherapy and long-term radiation-related side effects. Compared to RT alone, it does not look worse. However, whether chemoradiation is beneficial for these patients or not is not entirely clear because of limited data:

- Most of these studies examined women with stage I disease or II, limiting their applicability to these patients.
- Because of the disease's rarity, no randomized clinical trials have been performed.

In a study of 71 patients, 20 patients who received definitive RT concomitant chemotherapy and 51 who did not receive chemotherapy were evaluated. It was found that 3-year and overall survival were statistically significantly longer in the chemosensitive group, and disease-free survival rates were also longer in the chemotherapy group [45].

For patients with stage II to IV disease who are not considered candidates for chemoradiotherapy, RT (with intracavitary or interstitial therapy, depending on tumor thickness) is a reasonable alternative [39, 40, 46–49].

However, results after RT alone in advanced disease are not as good as in patients with stage I disease. In the same series from a single institution mentioned above, the two-year overall survival rate, regional control rate, and distant metastasis-free survival rate by stage were as follows [20]:

- Stage II – 92.3%, 64.7%, and 84.6%, respectively
- Stage III – 66.6%, 44.4%, and 50%
- Stage IV – 25%, 14.3% and 25%

In patients with advanced disease, surgery as a primary treatment modality is associated with poorer outcomes than chemoradiotherapy. For example, in a literature review, the mean five-year survival rates for patients with stage II, III, and IV disease after surgery were 52, 44, and 14%, respectively, with or without adjuvant radiotherapy [36].

In addition, negative margins in women with large or extensive lesions are usually challenging to achieve without sacrificing the bladder or rectum.

Neoadjuvant therapy: Radical surgery after neoadjuvant chemotherapy is a promising alternative to RT for these patients. However, we consider it mostly experimental until further data becomes available.

In a small prospective study of 11 patients with stage II disease who previously had three courses of 21 days of paclitaxel (175 mg/m^2) and cisplatin (75 mg/m^2) chemotherapy, the potential role of neoadjuvant therapy was demonstrated. 91% of these patients had a clinical response after neoadjuvant chemotherapy, and all were able to undergo surgical resection. The pathological complete response rate was 27% [50].

5. Complications

10–15% of patients with vaginal cancer will develop treatment-related complications [51]. These include rectovaginal or vesicovaginal fistulas, radiation cystitis or proctitis, rectal and vaginal strictures, and rarely vaginal necrosis. The proximity of the urethra, bladder, and rectum predisposes these structures to injury from surgery or radiation.

After radiation, women are advised to use a vaginal dilator to minimize the extent of vaginal stenosis. In general, we recommend that women start using the dilator one week after completing radiation and use it daily. Women who are sexually active regularly may need to use the dilator less frequently.

Women under 40 years of age who receive radiation for vaginal carcinoma are at higher risk for radiation-induced early menopause. In numerous ways, attempts to minimize the toxicity of radiation exposure by moving the ovaries to the back of the uterus or the lateral pelvic walls (oophoropexy) have been successful [52, 53]. It is recommended to perform oophoropexy in selected cases.

5.1 In case of recurrence

Recurrent patients may be candidates for surgery. However, for those who are not candidates for surgery for any reason, treatment options are rather limited because of the lack of prospective studies on this disease.

In patients with central recurrence and no other foci of disease, pelvic exenteration may be therapeutic with or without vaginal reconstruction [54–56]. Exenteration may also be considered in stage IVa patients, especially if a rectovaginal or vesicovaginal fistula is present.

Chemotherapy's role in recurrent or advanced vaginal cancer patients is unclear. Therefore, we administer chemotherapy to patients with recurrent vaginal cancer when there are no alternatives (e.g., surgery or radiotherapy [RT]) or when there is evidence of metastatic disease outside the pelvis. However, patients and providers should be aware that there is a lack of high-quality data to inform whether the benefits of treatment justify the toxicities associated with systemic chemotherapy. In the absence of clear benefits, these patients should be referred to palliative care when appropriate [57–60].

Cisplatin was recommended based on the experience of the Gynecological Oncology Group, which included 26 patients with advanced disease. Although the dose of cisplatin was sub-therapeutic by modern standards, these patients had insignificant activity (50 mg/m^2 every three weeks) [57]. Combination therapy with bleomycin, vincristine, mitomycin, and cisplatin also appears to be relatively ineffective in patients with advanced or recurrent disease, although it shows marked efficacy in early disease [58]. In patients with early-stage squamous vaginal carcinoma, anecdotal findings suggest an activity for carboplatin, a combination of vinblastine, bleomycin, and cisplatin, and irinotecan, as well as cisplatin [26, 59, 60]. However, a large series of these regimens is lacking to confirm activity in advanced disease.

6. Post treatment follow-up

The optimal surveillance strategy has not yet been determined, and clinical practice varies. We agree with the recommendations of the Society of Gynecological Oncology (SGO) [61]:

- Review of symptoms and physical examination:

- For low-risk disease (early stage, treated surgically only, no adjuvant therapy) - Every six months for the first two years and annually after that.

- For high-risk disease (advanced stage, treated with primary chemo/radiotherapy or surgery plus adjuvant therapy) - Every three months for the first two years, every six months for years 3 through 5, and annually after that.

- Cervical cytology (or vaginal cytology if the cervix has been removed) annually. However, the evaluations concluded that there is insufficient evidence to support the use of cytology to detect cancer recurrence but that it may help detect other neoplasms of the lower genital tract.

- Routine use of imaging studies is not recommended. Computed tomography (CT) and/or positron emission tomography (PET) should be performed if recurrence is suspected.

- If abnormalities are discovered during a physical examination, a vaginal colposcopy and biopsy are indicated.

Given the risk of multifocal vaginal illness and other human papillomavirus (HPV)-related diseases like cervical, vulvar, and anal neoplasia, these patients should also be screened for these diseases.

Following the therapy, sexual dysfunction and body image changes are prevalent and should be addressed during follow-up visits [62, 63].

7. Prognosis

The stage at presentation, which reflects the extent and depth of tumor penetration, is the most critical variable impacting the prognosis [13, 46, 49, 64–67]. Data from the United States National Cancer Database, for example, have shown an increased risk of death in women with stage II or higher disease and/or vaginal cancer with tumor size >4 cm (five-year survival 65% vs. 84 percent for tumors ≤4 cm), and the mortality rate for women with melanoma was 51% higher than for squamous cell carcinoma [67]. The lower survival rates in women with vaginal cancer compared with those with cervical or vulvar cancer may reflect the high rate of vaginal tumors diagnosed at an advanced stage and the potential for treatment complications that preclude aggressive treatment.

8. Conclusion

The stage at presentation, which indicates the degree and depth of tumor penetration, is the most critical variable impacting the prognosis in primary vaginal squamous cell cancer. The lower survival rates in women with primary vaginal cancer than those with cervical or vulvar cancer are related to a high diagnosis rate of advanced-stage vaginal tumors at baseline and potential treatment complications that preclude aggressive treatment.

Acknowledgements

We would like to express my gratitude to all those who helped me during the writing of this manuscript. Thanks to all the peer reviewers and editors for their opinions and suggestions.

Conflict of interest

The authors declare no conflict of interest.

Author details

Ferhat Cetin[1] and Özer Birge[2*]

1 Department of Gynecology and Obstetrics, Osmaniye State Hospital, Osmaniye, Turkey

2 Department of Gynecology and Obstetrics, Akdeniz University Hospital, Antalya, Turkey

*Address all correspondence to: ozbirge@gmail.com

References

[1] Siegel RL, Miller KD, Fuchs HE, Jemal A. Cancer statistics, 2021. CA: a Cancer Journal for Clinicians. 2021;**71**(1):7-33. DOI: 10.3322/caac.21654 Epub 2021 Jan 12. Erratum in: CA Cancer J Clin. 2021;71(4):359

[2] Dunn LJ, Napier JG. Primary carcinoma of the vagina. American Journal of Obstetrics and Gynecology. 1966;**96**(8):1112-1116. DOI: 10.1016/0002-9378(66)90519-9

[3] Way S. Vaginal metastases of carcinoma of the body of the uterus. The Journal of Obstetrics and Gynaecology of the British Empire. 1951;**58**(4):558-572. DOI: 10.1111/j.1471-0528.1951.tb04037.x

[4] Bergman F. Carcinoma of the ovary. A clinicopathological study of 86 autopsied cases with special reference to mode of spread. Acta Obstetricia et Gynecologica Scandinavica. 1966;**45**(2):211-231. DOI: 10.3109/00016346609158447

[5] Nerdrum TA. Vaginal metastasis of hypernephroma. Report of three cases. Acta Obstetricia et Gynecologica Scandinavica. 1966;**45**(4):515-524. DOI: 10.3109/00016346609158466

[6] Shah CA, Goff BA, Lowe K, Peters WA 3rd, Li CI. Factors affecting risk of mortality in women with vaginal cancer. Obstetrics and Gynecology. 2009;**113**(5):1038-1045. DOI: 10.1097/AOG.0b013e31819fe844

[7] Gadducci A, Fabrini MG, Lanfredini N, Sergiampietri C. Squamous cell carcinoma of the vagina: Natural history, treatment modalities and prognostic factors. Critical Reviews in Oncology/Hematology. 2015;**93**(3):211-224. DOI: 10.1016/j.critrevonc.2014.09.002

[8] Alemany L, Saunier M, Tinoco L, Quirós B, Alvarado-Cabrero I, Alejo M, et al. HPV VVAP study group. Large contribution of human papillomavirus in vaginal neoplastic lesions: A worldwide study in 597 samples. European Journal of Cancer. 2014;**50**(16):2846-2854. DOI: 10.1016/j.ejca.2014.07.018

[9] Daling JR, Madeleine MM, Schwartz SM, Shera KA, Carter JJ, McKnight B, et al. A population-based study of squamous cell vaginal cancer: HPV and cofactors. Gynecologic Oncology. 2002;**84**(2):263-270. DOI: 10.1006/gyno.2001.6502

[10] Madsen BS, Jensen HL, van den Brule AJ, Wohlfahrt J, Frisch M. Risk factors for invasive squamous cell carcinoma of the vulva and vagina--population-based case-control study in Denmark. International Journal of Cancer. 2008;**122**(12):2827-2834. DOI: 10.1002/ijc.23446

[11] Vinokurova S, Wentzensen N, Einenkel J, Klaes R, Ziegert C, Melsheimer P, et al. Clonal history of papillomavirus-induced dysplasia in the female lower genital tract. Journal of the National Cancer Institute. 2005;**97**(24):1816-1821. DOI: 10.1093/jnci/dji428

[12] Strander B, Andersson-Ellström A, Milsom I, Sparén P. Long term risk of invasive cancer after treatment for cervical intraepithelial neoplasia grade 3: Population based cohort study. BMJ. 2007;**335**(7629):1077. DOI: 10.1136/bmj.39363.471806.BE

[13] Kirkbride P, Fyles A, Rawlings GA, Manchul L, Levin W, Murphy KJ, et al. Carcinoma of the vagina--experience at the Princess Margaret hospital

(1974-1989). Gynecologic Oncology. 1995;**56**(3):435-443. DOI: 10.1006/gyno.1995.1077

[14] Choo YC, Anderson DG. Neoplasms of the vagina following cervical carcinoma. Gynecologic Oncology. 1982;**14**(1):125-132. DOI: 10.1016/0090-8258(82)90059-2

[15] Herbst AL, Ulfelder H, Poskanzer DC. Adenocarcinoma of the vagina. Association of maternal stilbestrol therapy with tumor appearance in young women. The New England Journal of Medicine. 1971;**284**(15):878-881. DOI: 10.1056/NEJM197104222841604

[16] Dunn LJ, Napier JG. Primary carcinoma of the vagina. American Journal of Obstetrics and Gynecology. 1966;**96**(8):1112-1116. DOI: 10.1016/0002-9378(66)90519-9

[17] Underwood PB Jr, Smith RT. Carcinoma of the vagina. Journal of the American Medical Association. 1971;**217**(1):46-52

[18] Pride GL, Schultz AE, Chuprevich TW, Buchler DA. Primary invasive squamous carcinoma of the vagina. Obstetrics and Gynecology. 1979;**53**(2):218-225

[19] Gallup DG, Talledo OE, Shah KJ, Hayes C. Invasive squamous cell carcinoma of the vagina: A 14-year study. Obstetrics and Gynecology. 1987;**69**(5):782-785

[20] Hiniker SM, Roux A, Murphy JD, Harris JP, Tran PT, Kapp DS, et al. Primary squamous cell carcinoma of the vagina: Prognostic factors, treatment patterns, and outcomes. Gynecologic Oncology. 2013;**131**(2):380-385. DOI: 10.1016/j.ygyno.2013.08.012

[21] Di Donato V, Bellati F, Fischetti M, Plotti F, Perniola G, Panici PB. Vaginal cancer. Critical Reviews in Oncology/Hematology. 2012;**81**(3):286-295. DOI: 10.1016/j.critrevonc.2011.04.004

[22] Taylor MB, Dugar N, Davidson SE, Carrington BM. Magnetic resonance imaging of primary vaginal carcinoma. Clinical Radiology. 2007;**62**(6):549-555. DOI: 10.1016/j.crad.2007.01.008

[23] Gardner CS, Sunil J, Klopp AH, Devine CE, Sagebiel T, Viswanathan C, et al. Primary vaginal cancer: Role of MRI in diagnosis, staging and treatment. The British Journal of Radiology. 2015;**88**(1052):20150033. DOI: 10.1259/bjr.20150033

[24] Lamoreaux WT, Grigsby PW, Dehdashti F, Zoberi I, Powell MA, Gibb RK, et al. FDG-PET evaluation of vaginal carcinoma. International Journal of Radiation Oncology, Biology, Physics. 2005;**62**(3):733-737. DOI: 10.1016/j.ijrobp.2004.12.011

[25] MacKinnon R, Elmezzi K, Phippen N. Vaginal dermoid cyst. American Journal of Obstetrics and Gynecology. 2021;**225**(3):337-338. DOI: 10.1016/j.ajog.2021.03.010

[26] Creasman WT, Phillips JL, Menck HR. The National Cancer data base report on cancer of the vagina. Cancer. 1998;**83**(5):1033-1040

[27] Ikenberg H, Runge M, Göppinger A, Pfleiderer A. Human papillomavirus DNA in invasive carcinoma of the vagina. Obstetrics and Gynecology. 1990;**76** (3 Pt 1):432-438

[28] Isaacs JH. Verrucous carcinoma of the female genital tract. Gynecologic Oncology. 1976;**4**(3):259-269. DOI: 10.1016/0090-8258(76)90031-7

[29] Shrivastava SB, Agrawal G, Mittal M, Mishra P. Management of vaginal cancer. Reviews on Recent Clinical Trials. 2015;**10**(4):289-297. DOI: 10.2174/1574887110666150923112958

[30] FIGO Committee on Gynecologic Oncology. Current FIGO staging for cancer of the vagina, fallopian tube, ovary, and gestational trophoblastic neoplasia. International Journal of Gynaecology and Obstetrics. 2009;**105**(1):3-4. DOI: 10.1016/j.ijgo.2008.12.015

[31] Benedet JL, Bender H, Jones H 3rd, Ngan HY, Pecorelli S. FIGO staging classifications and clinical practice guidelines in the management of gynecologic cancers. FIGO Committee on Gynecologic Oncology. International Journal of Gynaecology and Obstetrics. 2000;**70**(2):209-262

[32] Hacker NF, Eifel PJ. Vaginal cancer. In: Berek JS, Hacker NF, editors. Berek and Hacker's Gynecologic Oncology. 7th ed. USA: Kluwer; 2021. pp. 547-561. ISBN:978-1-97-514264-3

[33] Lian J, Dundas G, Carlone M, Ghosh S, Pearcey R. Twenty-year review of radiotherapy for vaginal cancer: An institutional experience. Gynecologic Oncology. 2008;**111**(2):298-306. DOI: 10.1016/j.ygyno.2008.07.007

[34] Stock RG, Chen AS, Seski J. A 30-year experience in the management of primary carcinoma of the vagina: Analysis of prognostic factors and treatment modalities. Gynecologic Oncology. 1995;**56**(1):45-52. DOI: 10.1006/gyno.1995.1008

[35] Hacker NF, Eifel PJ, van der Velden J. Cancer of the vagina. International Journal of Gynaecology and Obstetrics. 2012;**119**(Suppl. 2):S97-S99. DOI: 10.1016/S0020-7292(12)60022-8

[36] Tjalma WA, Monaghan JM, de Barros LA, Naik R, Nordin AJ, Weyler JJ. The role of surgery in invasive squamous carcinoma of the vagina. Gynecologic Oncology. 2001;**81**(3):360-365. DOI: 10.1006/gyno.2001.6171

[37] Orton A, Boothe D, Williams N, Buchmiller T, Huang YJ, Suneja G, et al. Brachytherapy improves survival in primary vaginal cancer. Gynecologic Oncology. 2016;**141**(3):501-506. DOI: 10.1016/j.ygyno.2016.03.011

[38] Stock RG, Mychalczak B, Armstrong JG, Curtin JP, Harrison LB. The importance of brachytherapy technique in the management of primary carcinoma of the vagina. International Journal of Radiation Oncology, Biology, Physics. 1992;**24**(4):747-753. DOI: 10.1016/0360-3016(92)90724-v

[39] Tran PT, Su Z, Lee P, Lavori P, Husain A, Teng N, et al. Prognostic factors for outcomes and complications for primary squamous cell carcinoma of the vagina treated with radiation. Gynecologic Oncology. 2007;**105**(3):641-649. DOI: 10.1016/j.ygyno.2007.01.033

[40] Frank SJ, Jhingran A, Levenback C, Eifel PJ. Definitive radiation therapy for squamous cell carcinoma of the vagina. International Journal of Radiation Oncology, Biology, Physics. 2005;**62**(1):138-147. DOI: 10.1016/j.ijrobp.2004.09.032

[41] Grigsby PW. Vaginal cancer. Current Treatment Options in Oncology. 2002;**3**(2):125-130. DOI: 10.1007/s11864-002-0058-4

[42] Dalrymple JL, Russell AH, Lee SW, Scudder SA, Leiserowitz GS, Kinney WK, et al. Chemoradiation for primary invasive squamous carcinoma

of the vagina. International Journal of Gynecological Cancer. 2004;**14**(1):110-117. DOI: 10.1111/j.1048-891x.2004.014066.x

[43] Roberts WS, Hoffman MS, Kavanagh JJ, Fiorica JV, Greenberg H, Finan MA, et al. Further experience with radiation therapy and concomitant intravenous chemotherapy in advanced carcinoma of the lower female genital tract. Gynecologic Oncology. 1991;**43**(3):233-236. DOI: 10.1016/0090-8258(91)90026-2

[44] Samant R, Lau B, Choan E, Le T, Tam T. Primary vaginal cancer treated with concurrent chemoradiation using Cis-platinum. International Journal of Radiation Oncology, Biology, Physics. 2007;**69**(3):746-750. DOI: 10.1016/j.ijrobp.2007.04.015

[45] Miyamoto DT, Viswanathan AN. Concurrent chemoradiation for vaginal cancer. PLoS One. 2013;**8**(6):e65048. DOI: 10.1371/journal.pone.0065048

[46] Tewari KS, Cappuccini F, Puthawala AA, Kuo JV, Burger RA, Monk BJ, et al. Primary invasive carcinoma of the vagina: Treatment with interstitial brachytherapy. Cancer. 2001;**91**(4):758-770. DOI: 10.1002/1097-0142(20010215)91:4<758::aid-cncr1062>3.0.co;2-u

[47] Reddy S, Saxena VS, Reddy S, Lee MS, Yordan EL, Graham JE, et al. Results of radiotherapeutic management of primary carcinoma of the vagina. International Journal of Radiation Oncology, Biology, Physics. 1991;**21**(4):1041-1044. DOI: 10.1016/0360-3016(91)90747-r

[48] Spirtos NM, Doshi BP, Kapp DS, Teng N. Radiation therapy for primary squamous cell carcinoma of the vagina: Stanford University experience. Gynecologic Oncology. 1989;**35**(1):20-26. DOI: 10.1016/0090-8258(89)90004-8

[49] Perez CA, Grigsby PW, Garipagaoglu M, Mutch DG, Lockett MA. Factors affecting long-term outcome of irradiation in carcinoma of the vagina. International Journal of Radiation Oncology, Biology, Physics. 1999;**44**(1):37-45. DOI: 10.1016/s0360-3016(98)00530-6

[50] Benedetti Panici P, Bellati F, Plotti F, Di Donato V, Antonilli M, Perniola G, et al. Neoadjuvant chemotherapy followed by radical surgery in patients affected by vaginal carcinoma. Gynecologic Oncology. 2008;**111**(2):307-311. DOI: 10.1016/j.ygyno.2008.07.005

[51] Rubin SC, Young J, Mikuta JJ. Squamous carcinoma of the vagina: Treatment, complications, and long-term follow-up. Gynecologic Oncology. 1985;**20**(3):346-353. DOI: 10.1016/0090-8258(85)90216-1

[52] Chambers SK, Chambers JT, Kier R, Peschel RE. Sequelae of lateral ovarian transposition in irradiated cervical cancer patients. International Journal of Radiation Oncology, Biology, Physics. 1991;**20**(6):1305-1308. DOI: 10.1016/0360-3016(91)90242-v

[53] Damewood MD, Hesla HS, Lowen M, Schultz MJ. Induction of ovulation and pregnancy following lateral oophoropexy for Hodgkin's disease. International Journal of Gynaecology and Obstetrics. 1990;**33**(4):369-371. DOI: 10.1016/0020-7292(90)90524-o

[54] Al-Kurdi M, Monaghan JM. Thirty-two years experience in management of primary tumours of the vagina. British Journal of Obstetrics and Gynaecology. 1981;**88**(11):1145-1150. DOI: 10.1111/j.1471-0528.1981.tb01770.x

[55] Berek JS, Hacker NF, Lagasse LD. Vaginal reconstruction performed simultaneously with pelvic exenteration. Obstetrics and Gynecology. 1984; **63**(3):318-323

[56] Benson C, Soisson AP, Carlson J, Culbertson G, Hawley-Bowland C, Richards F. Neovaginal reconstruction with a rectus abdominis myocutaneous flap. Obstetrics and Gynecology. 1993;**81**(5 (Pt 2)):871-875

[57] Thigpen JT, Blessing JA, Homesley HD, Berek JS, Creasman WT. Phase II trial of cisplatin in advanced or recurrent cancer of the vagina: A Gynecologic oncology group study. Gynecologic Oncology. 1986;**23**(1):101-104. DOI: 10.1016/0090-8258(86)90121-6

[58] Belinson JL, Stewart JA, Richards AL, McClure M. Bleomycin, vincristine, mitomycin-C, and cisplatin in the management of gynecological squamous cell carcinomas. Gynecologic Oncology. 1985;**20**(3):387-393. DOI: 10.1016/0090-8258(85)90220-3

[59] Umesaki N, Kawamura N, Tsujimura A, Ichimura T, Tanaka T, Ogita S. Stage II vaginal cancer responding to chemotherapy with irinotecan and cisplatin: A case report. Oncology Reports. 1999;**6**(1):123-125. DOI: 10.3892/or.6.1.123

[60] Kim DS, Moon H, Hwang YY, Park MI. Histologic disappearance of locally advanced vaginal cancer after combination chemotherapy. Gynecologic Oncology. 1990;**38**(1):144-145. DOI: 10.1016/0090-8258(90)90029-k

[61] Salani R, Backes FJ, Fung MF, Holschneider CH, Parker LP, Bristow RE, et al. Posttreatment surveillance and diagnosis of recurrence in women with gynecologic malignancies: Society of Gynecologic Oncologists recommendations. American Journal of Obstetrics and Gynecology. 2011;**204**(6):466-478. DOI: 10.1016/j.ajog.2011.03.008

[62] Andreasson B, Moth I, Jensen SB, Bock JE. Sexual function and somatopsychic reactions in vulvectomy-operated women and their partners. Acta Obstetricia et Gynecologica Scandinavica. 1986;**65**(1):7-10. DOI: 10.3109/00016348609158221

[63] Green MS, Naumann RW, Elliot M, Hall JB, Higgins RV, Grigsby JH. Sexual dysfunction following vulvectomy. Gynecologic Oncology. 2000;**77**(1):73-77. DOI: 10.1006/gyno.2000.5745

[64] Nori D, Hilaris BS, Stanimir G, Lewis JL Jr. Radiation therapy of primary vaginal carcinoma. International Journal of Radiation Oncology, Biology, Physics. 1983;**9**(10):1471-1475. DOI: 10.1016/0360-3016(83)90320-6

[65] Brady LW, Perez CA, Bedwinek JM. Failure patterns in gynecologic cancer. International Journal of Radiation Oncology, Biology, Physics. 1986;**12**(4):549-557. DOI: 10.1016/0360-3016(86)90062-3

[66] Hellman K, Lundell M, Silfverswärd C, Nilsson B, Hellström AC, Frankendal B. Clinical and histopathologic factors related to prognosis in primary squamous cell carcinoma of the vagina. International Journal of Gynecological Cancer. 2006;**16**(3):1201-1211. DOI: 10.1111/j.1525-1438.2006.00520.x

[67] Beller U, Sideri M, Maisonneuve P, Benedet JL, Heintz AP, Ngan HY, et al. Carcinoma of the vagina. Journal of Epidemiology and Biostatistics. 2001;**6**(1):141-152

Chapter 2

Squamous Cell Carcinoma of Bladder

Ferhat Cetin and Özer Birge

Abstract

Urinary bladder tumors are the second most common malignancy of the urinary system. In 2012, the global age-standardized incidence rate (per 100,000 person/years) was reported as 9.0 for men and 2.2 for women. Usually, bladder cancers are seen in middle and old-aged people. In the United States, the average age for getting a diagnosis was 72 years. It was reported that 90% of newly diagnosed patients were above 60 years and rarely below 35 years. Bladder tumors relapse approximately 50–75% within 5 years after diagnosis, and progressions occur in 10–20% of them. While the five-year survival rate of organ-confined disease is 94%, the survival rates of locally invasive and metastatic tumors varied between 6 and 49%. Most of the bladder urothelial carcinomas diagnosed in patients under 40 years of age are low-grade and stage I, and the 5-year survival rate is around 97%.

Keywords: bladder, urinary system, squamous cell carcinoma

1. Introduction

Bladder cancer is the most frequent genitourinary malignancy in both men and women. They are divided into two groups—urothelial and nonurothelial.

2. Anatomy

The bladder is located in the midline just behind the pubic bone. The bladder is separated from the pubic bone by the retropubic space, also known as the Retzius space, including the Santorini venous plexus. The symphysis pubis, laterally the pelvic side-walls, posteriorly and inferiorly the lower uterine segment, anterior cervix, and vagina are the bladder's boundaries. The obliterated umbilical artery and urachus correspond to the upper border of the bladder. The urachus connects the developing bladder to the umbilicus in the fetus. After birth, the urachus curves into the median umbilical ligament, which connects the apex of the bladder to the anterior abdominal wall. Sometimes, the urachus remains patent. The bladder dome is located next to the anterior abdominal wall's parietal peritoneum. The bladder is pushed into the vesicouterine space by the peritoneum below. The bladder's thick parts are retroperitoneal. The bladder is an organ that has the ability to expand. When empty, it has the shape of a pyramid. The tip points to the pubic bone. It becomes a sphere when it is full, with a capacity of about 400–500 cc in a healthy adult individual, and it changes from a pelvic to an abdominal organ in this state. When the dome is completely filled, the dome's structure becomes thinner than the dome's other parts. As a result, emptying the bladder with the aid of a catheter before beginning pelvic surgery can assist in preventing bladder injuries. The upper dome and lower floor are present in the bladder. The bladder floor, which comprises the trigone and detrusor ring, is located directly on the anterior wall of the vagina. Thickening of the detrusor muscle is a thickening that does not change directly with bladder filling. The area between the two ureteral orifices and the internal urethral meatus is known as the bladder trigone. The two ureteral orifices and the internal urethral meatus are 3 cm apart. The intraurethral ridge is a rise in the trigone between the ureteral orifices [1].

The bladder wall is made up of four layers:

a. Urothelium

The urothelium is the bladder's innermost layer, consisting of transitional epithelial cells. Bladder cancer originates in the urothelial layer.

b. Lamina propria

A thin basement membrane separates the lamina propria (subepithelial connective tissue) from the urothelium. This layer consists of rich connective tissue containing vascular and neuronal structures. Thin, smooth muscle fibers may be present in the middle of this layer, partially or as a separate layer, along with the vascular plexus. This area is also called muscular mucosa.

c. Muscularis propria

The muscularis propria (detrusor muscle) are thick, interlocking, irregular muscle bundles surrounding the lamina propria. When the bladder contracts, the detrusor muscle's plexiform structure is ideal for reducing all lumen dimensions. Small muscle fibers in the lamina propria (muscularis mucosa) described above can be confused with this layer in small biopsies, potentially leading to incorrect tumor staging. The lamina propria and/or muscularis propria may include adipose tissue. Therefore, the presence of a tumor in adipose tissue does not always indicate extravesical spread.

d. Serosa (adventitia)

It is the name for the perivesical adipose tissue outside the muscularis propria [1, 2].

The superior and inferior vesical arteries, which arise from the anterior branch of the internal iliac artery, give blood to the bladder. The pelvic and hypogastric nerve plexuses' parasympathetic and sympathetic autonomic fibers supply bladder innervation [1].

3. Epidemiology

Nonurothelial bladder cancer makes up fewer than 5% of all bladder tumors [3]. About 90% of nonurothelial bladder cancers are epithelial in origin. Most of them are squamous cell carcinomas; other rare types are adenocarcinomas and small cell carcinomas. Non-epithelial tumors include sarcomas, carcinosarcomas, paragangliomas, melanomas, and lymphomas.

4. Pathogenesis and risk factors

The pathogenesis of nonurothelial bladder cancers is not fully understood. The presence of chronic infection and metaplasia development are believed to be crucial factors in tumorigenesis. Alternative hypotheses include the development of nonurothelial bladder cancers from pre-existing urothelial (transitional cell) carcinomas undergoing metaplasia [4] and tumor growth from multipotent stem cells in the bladder.

Chronic infection and inflammation cause tissue metaplasia, resulting in the development of either squamous epithelium and leukoplakia or mucous and glandular epithelium. The factors that cause neoplastic transformation, on the other hand, are unknown.

- Squamous cell carcinomas are frequently associated with squamous metaplasia and occur in 16–28% of leukoplakia patients [5, 6].

- Adenocarcinoma has been linked to two models of metaplasia. Invagination of hyperplastic epithelial buds into the lamina propria causes cystitis cystica, which can progress to metaplasia and cystitis glandularis and is linked to vesical adenocarcinoma. Hyperplasia of epithelial mother cells is shown in a second pattern, but there is no invagination into the lamina propria.

Both non-schistosomal and schistosomal bladder cancer are associated with chronic urinary tract infections (UTIs). Infection may play a role in the development of bladder cancer through a variety of mechanisms, including:

- Predisposition to metaplasia is the first step in carcinogenesis.

- Gram-negative bacteria, such as *Escherichia coli* and *Proteus mirabilis*, create nitrosamines, which are extremely carcinogenic metabolites. Carcinogenesis results from the formation of DNA adducts and possibly by other mechanisms [7–12].

- Inflammatory cells' production of reactive oxygen species in response to infection causes DNA damage and the activation of additional carcinogens.

5. Clinical presentation

Patients with nonurothelial bladder cancer often have painless hematuria (visible or microscopic), but irritating urination symptoms (frequency, urgency, and dysuria) may be the initial indicator, similar to urothelial carcinomas.

Nonurothelial bladder cancers have a variety of less common presentations, including:

- Mucusuria has been described in bladder adenocarcinomas and is more common in urachal adenocarcinomas than in non-urachal adenocarcinomas.

- The presence of an abdominal mass is more common in urachal adenocarcinoma compared to in non-urachal adenocarcinoma.

6. Diagnostic evaluation

Cystoscopy is the gold standard for diagnosing a patient with a suspected bladder neoplasm, and cystoscopic biopsy typically gives tissue for a definite diagnosis. Compared to urothelial cancers, non-urothelial tumors are more likely to be muscle-invasive at diagnosis and more likely to be staged at the time of surgery because precise pathological staging is available. Therefore, as a group, non-urothelial tumors occur at a more advanced stage and contribute to a worse prognosis compared to urothelial cancers [13]. However, an interesting observation is that urachal cancers tend to have a better prognosis at presentation than urothelial cancers at a similar stage (**Table 1**) [14].

Primary tumor (T)	
T category	**T criterion**
TX	Primary tumor unknown
T0	No evidence of primary tumor
Ta	Noninvasive papillary tumor
Tis	Carcinoma *in situ*: "Flat tumor"
T1	Invasive to the lamina propria
T2	Invasive into the muscularis propria
pT2a	Invasive into the superficial muscularis propria
pT2b	Invasive into the deep muscularis propria
T3	Invasive perivesical adipose tissue
pT3a	Microscopic
pT3b	Macroscopic
T4	Extravesical tumor invasive of either the prostatic stroma, seminal vesicle, uterus, vagina, pelvic wall, or abdominal wall
T4a	Extravesical tumor invading the prostatic stroma, seminal vesicle, uterus, and vagina
T4b	Extravesical tumor of the pelvic wall, invasive into the abdominal wall
Regional lymph nodes (N)	
N category	**N criterion**
NX	Lymph node metastasis unknown
N0	No lymph node metastases
N1	Single regional lymph node metastasis in the true pelvis (perivesical, obturator, internal iliac, external iliac, or sacral lymph node)
N2	Multiple regional lymph node metastases in the true pelvis (perivesical, obturator, internal iliac, external iliac, or sacral lymph nodes)
N3	Common iliac lymph node metastasis
Distant metastasis (M)	
M category	**M criterion**
M0	No distant metastases
M1	There is distant metastasis
M1a	Distant metastasis limited beyond the common iliac

Distant metastasis (M)			
M category	**M criterion**		
M1b	Presence of distant metastases without lymph node metastasis		
Prognostic staging groups			
When T is like this	**When N is like this**	**When M is like this**	**The staging group goes like this**
Ta	N0	M0	0a
Tis	N0	M0	0is
T1	N0	M0	I
T2a	N0	M0	II
T2b	N0	M0	II
T3a, T3b, T4a	N0	M0	IIIA
T1-T4a	N1	M0	IIIA
T1-T4a	N2, N3	M0	IIIB
T4b	Any N	M0	IVA
Any T	Any N	M1a	IVA
Any T	Any N	M1b	IVB

Table 1.
AJCC cancer staging 2017.

7. Overview of the treatment approach

The treatment of nonurothelial bladder tumors is mainly based on retrospective series and small trials due to their rarity and heterogeneity. As a result, the approach to patients with urothelial bladder cancer is frequently used to estimate treatment.

Cystectomy is the primary treatment for patients with localized illness. This should include a lymph node dissection with radical cystectomy for individuals with squamous carcinoma, adenocarcinoma, or schistosomal bladder cancer (regardless of histology).

Nonurothelial carcinomas of the bladder, ureter, or renal pelvis are not recommended for preoperative or postoperative chemotherapy because they are less responsive to chemotherapy than urothelial carcinomas and were not included in the phase III trials.

Although radiation therapy (RT) before cystectomy may play a role in schistosomal bladder cancer, it is not a standard treatment approach for other bladder tumors [15, 16]. There are no high-quality data on the role of chemotherapy and/or RT as adjuvant therapy.

Palliative care, RT, or chemotherapy are options for patients with advanced nonurothelial bladder cancer who are not candidates for surgery, including those with metastatic disease. Such patients should participate in clinical trials whenever possible. However, a trial of chemotherapy is reasonable in patients who are candidates for chemotherapy and are in good performance status. When deciding on treatment, it should be kept in mind that there are no prospective data that provide information on the benefits of treatment compared with the risks associated with treatment.

Because trials for certain groups of nonurothelial carcinomas are not common, these patients are often candidates for early phase clinical trials and "basket studies" that allow enrollment of tumors with specific mutations that are considered "vulnerable" to the drug being offered. According to case reports, nonurothelial malignancies may react to targeted agents found by molecular profiling techniques, such as next-generation sequencing [17, 18]. Patients with potentially actionable mutations in their tumors should be included in clinical studies that capture molecular, response, and outcome data prospectively whenever possible [19, 20].

8. Squamous cell carcinoma

In North America and Europe, squamous cell carcinoma accounts for 3 to 5% of bladder cancers and 75% of bladder cancers in areas where *Schistosoma haematobium* infection is endemic.

Risk factors associated with the development of squamous cell carcinoma include chronic or recurrent urinary tract infections (UTIs), bladder stones, pelvic radiotherapy (RT), previous intravesical Bacillus Calmette-Guerin (BCG) therapy, and prolonged cyclophosphamide treatment, especially when complicated by hemorrhagic cystitis, in addition to schistosome infection [3]. Although smoking raises the risk of squamous cell carcinoma [21, 22], an observational study with long-term follow-up reveals that patients with pure squamous cell carcinoma are more likely to be female and have never smoked than patients with urothelial carcinoma [23]. In some studies, chronic indwelling catheters have also been associated with an increased risk of squamous cell carcinoma, while the relationship is controversial.

Although the design of these studies and the prevalence of squamous cell cancer and adenocarcinoma in these patients may have precluded a statistically significant result, two large population-based studies in patients with spinal cord injury did not find an increased risk of bladder cancer [24, 25]. However, muscle invasion was more common in bladder cancer detected in patients with neurogenic bladder, and researchers preferred intermittent catheterization to indwelling catheters [25]. Although some investigators have recommended regular screening cystoscopies for patients with spinal cord injury, no studies have proved a benefit of screening, perhaps because of the extremely low incidence of cancer in these patients [26, 27].

Surgery is the primary treatment for squamous cell carcinoma. Preoperative RT is appropriate, especially when complete resection is possible due to suspected locally advanced disease.

The role of surgery is supported by observational and retrospective data. In a study of 1422 patients diagnosed with bladder cancer between 1988 and 2003, the two-year all-cause mortality rate following cystectomy ranged from 11% in men with stage I disease to 72% in men with stage IV disease, according to the results of a Surveillance, Epidemiology, and Final Results (SEER) database analysis [28]. Squamous cell carcinoma histology was statistically associated with worse prognosis outcomes than urothelial bladder cancer histology when age, gender, race, and starting treatment were classified equally for both groups.

The tendency for local recurrence of bladder squamous cell carcinoma after radical cystectomy provides the rationale for preoperative or postoperative RT with or without radiosensitizing chemotherapy. Unfortunately, due to the small number of patients included, bias in patient selection, and treatment heterogeneity, the quality of available data is limited.

Because of the risk of intestinal toxicity and the difficulty of determining an appropriate RT treatment region after bladder removal, preoperative RT is preferable to postoperative therapy in such cases. However, several retrospective case series have indicated potential benefits of adjuvant or neoadjuvant RT [29–32]. There has only been one prospective study on schistosomiasis infection, and the results may not apply to non-schistosomal squamous cell carcinoma.

Postoperative RT is a reasonable option for patients with locally progressed squamous cell bladder cancer following radical cystectomy unsuitable for or refusing adjuvant chemotherapy. New evidence supports its usage in patients with surgical margins that are positive [33]. In preliminary results of a randomized phase III trial of 123 patients with locally advanced bladder cancer (51% with urothelial carcinoma and 49% with squamous cell carcinoma or other carcinomas) after radical cystectomy versus adjuvant chemotherapy, RT improved local control (two-year local disease-free survival 92% vs. 69%, HR 0.28, 95% CI 0.10–0.82) [34]. The two treatment arms had similar disease-free survival, distant metastasis-free survival, and overall survival. Similar results were seen in a subgroup of patients with urothelial carcinoma [35].

Radiation combined with radiosensitizing chemotherapy (as is done for squamous cell carcinoma of the head and neck, anus, and uterine cervix) is a reasonable approach for patients with locally advanced, unresectable squamous cell carcinoma of the bladder, especially since these tumors tend to be locally aggressive. However, there are few forward-looking data to guide treatment.

Data from the phase III study BC2001 demonstrate efficacy for fluorouracil and mitomycin given with RT compared to RT alone in patients with high-grade muscular-invasive bladder cancer, who tend to have improved local and regional control and better survival [36]. Only 2.7% of patients in this trial had adenocarcinoma or squamous cell carcinoma, and there was no difference in outcomes compared to urothelial cancer. In patients with squamous cell carcinoma of the anus, a very comparable regimen is effective and well-tolerated; thus, extrapolation to squamous cell cancer of the bladder may be reasonable, especially in patients who are poor candidates for platinum-containing chemotherapy [37, 38].

Limited data suggest that squamous cell carcinoma tends to be locally advanced or worse at diagnosis and relatively resistant to chemotherapies used for metastatic urothelial carcinoma [23, 39–41]. We prefer that these patients participate in a prospective clinical trial in view of these results. The encouraging results of immunotherapy with T-cell checkpoint inhibitors using atezolizumab or pembrolizumab in advanced urothelial carcinoma previously treated with platinum-based therapy [42, 43], as well as the results of immunotherapy in patients with squamous cell carcinoma of the lung and head and neck tumors, support the inclusion of patients with squamous cell carcinoma of the urinary bladder in clinical trials, and we, therefore, continue to seek such trials for these patients [42, 43].

Treatment regimens used to treat metastatic urothelial cancer could be tried in the absence of a clinical trial. Based on phase II trial data in which six patients with bladder squamous cell carcinoma were treated with satisfactory results, similar to urothelial cancer patients in the same study, we recommend the combination of carboplatin, gemcitabine, and paclitaxel [44]. The experience from this trial is reproducible in our clinical practice for advanced squamous cell carcinoma of the bladder.

9. Prognosis

It is unclear whether nonurothelial bladder cancers have a worse prognosis, especially after controlling for stage and grade. After controlling for gender, stage, and grade, a multi-institutional study of 1131 consecutive patients (including 1042 with urothelial carcinoma and 89 with nonurothelial bladder cancer) found no differences in five-year survival following radical cystectomy [45].

10. Conclusion

Urothelial and nonurothelial bladder cancers are the two types of bladder cancer. Nonurothelial bladder cancers are further divided into epithelial and non-epithelial. Squamous cell carcinomas, adenocarcinomas, and small cell (neuroendocrine) tumors are epithelial cancers that account for around 90% of these cancers. Non-epithelial cancers are rare and include sarcomas, carcinosarcomas, paragangliomas, melanomas, and lymphomas. The pathogenesis of nonurothelial bladder cancers is not fully understood. The presence of chronic infection and inflammation, as well as the development of metaplasia, are regarded to be important factors in tumorigenesis. Like urothelial carcinomas, nonurothelial bladder carcinomas often present with hematuria and bladder irritation. Mucusuria has been described in bladder adenocarcinomas and is more common in urachal types than in non-urachal adenocarcinomas. The presence of an abdominal mass may also suggest a diagnosis of adenocarcinoma of the urinary bladder. Infection with *Schistosoma haematobium* is associated with squamous cell carcinoma, urothelial carcinoma, and adenocarcinoma of the bladder. Nonurothelial bladder cancers account for 80% of bladder cancer cases in areas where such infections are endemic. We recommend surgery for most patients with non-metastatic, nonurothelial bladder cancer. Adjuvant therapy does not have a defined role in most of these patients, although some patients may benefit from neoadjuvant or adjuvant radiotherapy, and patients with schistosomal bladder cancer may benefit from adjuvant chemoradiation. We recommend palliative treatment for patients with advanced bladder cancer who are not candidates for surgery. However, a trial of chemotherapy is reasonable in patients who are candidates for chemotherapy and are in good performance status. When deciding on treatment, it should be kept in mind that there are no prospective data that provide information on the benefits of treatment compared with the risks associated with treatment. In patients with non-epithelial, nonurothelial bladder cancer, in the absence of better evidence, we use the most appropriate treatments for these tumor types when they occur elsewhere. However, it is important to ensure that metastatic disease is excluded.

Acknowledgements

We would like to express our gratitude to all those who helped us during the writing of this manuscript. Thanks to all the peer reviewers and editors for their opinions and suggestions.

Conflict of interest

The authors declare no conflict of interest.

Author details

Ferhat Cetin[1*] and Özer Birge[2]

1 Department of Gynaecology and Obstetrics, Osmaniye State Hospital, Osmaniye, Turkey

2 Department of Gynaecology and Obstetrics, Akdeniz University Hospital, Antalya, Turkey

*Address all correspondence to: ferhat_cetin@hotmail.com

References

[1] Rahn DD, Bleich AT, Wai CY, Roshanravan SM, Wieslander CK, Schaffer JI, et al. Anatomic relationships of the distal third of the pelvic ureter, trigone, and urethra in unembalmed female cadavers. American Journal of Obstetrics and Gynecology. 2007;**197**(6):668.e1-668.e4. DOI: 10.1016/j.ajog.2007.08.068

[2] Reuter VE. The pathology of bladder cancer. Urology. 2006;**67**(3 Suppl 1): 11-17; discussion 17-18. DOI: 10.1016/j.urology.2006.01.037

[3] Dahm P, Gschwend JE. Malignant non-urothelial neoplasms of the urinary bladder: A review. European Urology. 2003;**44**(6):672-681. DOI: 10.1016/s0302-2838(03)00416-0

[4] Kunze E. Histogenesis of nonurothelial carcinomas in the human and rat urinary bladder. Experimental and Toxicologic Pathology. 1998;**50**(4-6):341-355. DOI: 10.1016/S0940-2993(98)80015-8

[5] Ozbey I, Aksoy Y, Polat O, Biçgi O, Demirel A. Squamous metaplasia of the bladder: Findings in 14 patients and review of the literature. International Urology and Nephrology. 1999;**31**(4): 457-461. DOI: 10.1023/a:1007107110222

[6] Khan MS, Thornhill JA, Gaffney E, LoftusB,ButlerMR.Keratinisingsquamous metaplasia of the bladder: Natural history and rationalization of management based on review of 54 years experience. European Urology. 2002;**42**(5):469-474. DOI: 10.1016/s0302-2838(02)00358-5

[7] El-Merzabani MM, El-Aaser AA, Zakhary NI. A study on the aetiological factors of bilharzial bladder cancer in Egypt--1. Nitrosamines and their precursors in urine. European Journal of Cancer. 1979;**15**(3):287-291. DOI: 10.1016/0014-2964(79)90039-2

[8] Radomski JL, Greenwald D, Hearn WL, Block NL, Woods FM. Nitrosamine formation in bladder infections and its role in the etiology of bladder cancer. The Journal of Urology. 1978;**120**(1):48-50. DOI: 10.1016/s0022-5347(17)57035-4

[9] Bartsch H, Montesano R. Relevance of nitrosamines to human cancer. Carcinogenesis. 1984;**5**(11):1381-1393. DOI: 10.1093/carcin/5.11.1381

[10] Wogan GN, Hecht SS, Felton JS, Conney AH, Loeb LA. Environmental and chemical carcinogenesis. Seminars in Cancer Biology. 2004;**14**(6):473-486. DOI: 10.1016/j.semcancer.2004.06.010

[11] Oliveira PA, Colaco A, De la Cruz PLF, Lopes C. Experimental bladder carcinogenesis-rodent models. Experimental Oncology. 2006;**28**(1):2-11

[12] El-Mosalamy H, Salman TM, Ashmawey AM, Osama N. Role of chronic *E. coli* infection in the process of bladder cancer—an experimental study. Infectious Agents and Cancer. 2012;7(1):19. DOI: 10.1186/1750-9378-7-19

[13] Deuker M, Martin T, Stolzenbach F, Rosiello G, Collà Ruvolo C, Nocera L, et al. Bladder cancer: A comparison between non-urothelial variant histology and urothelial carcinoma across all stages and treatment modalities. Clinical Genitourinary Cancer. 2021;**19**(1):60-68.e1. DOI: 10.1016/j.clgc.2020.07.011. Epub 2020 Jul 18

[14] Cohen AJ, Packiam V, Nottingham C, Steinberg G, Smith ND, Patel S.

Upstaging of nonurothelial histology in bladder cancer at the time of surgical treatment in the National Cancer Data Base. Urologic Oncology. 2017;**35**(1):34.e1-34.e8. DOI: 10.1016/j.urolonc.2016.08.002. Epub 2016 Sep 1

[15] Ghoneim MA, Ashamallah AK, Awaad HK, Whitmore WF Jr. Randomized trial of cystectomy with or without preoperative radiotherapy for carcinoma of the bilharzial bladder. The Journal of Urology. 1985;**134**(2):266-268. DOI: 10.1016/s0022-5347(17)47119-9

[16] Awwad H, El-Baki HA, El-Bolkainy N, Burgers M, El-Badawy S, Mansour M, et al. Pre-operative irradiation of T3-carcinoma in bilharzial bladder: A comparison between hyperfractionation and conventional fractionation. International Journal of Radiation Oncology, Biology, Physics. 1979;**5**(6):787-794. DOI: 10.1016/0360-3016(79)90062-2

[17] Collazo-Lorduy A, Castillo-Martin M, Wang L, Patel V, Iyer G, Jordan E, et al. Urachal carcinoma shares genomic alterations with colorectal carcinoma and may respond to epidermal growth factor inhibition. European Urology. 2016;**70**(5):771-775. DOI: 10.1016/j.eururo.2016.04.037. Epub 2016 May 10

[18] Loh KP, Mondo E, Hansen EA, Sievert L, Fung C, Sahasrabudhe DM, et al. Targeted therapy based on tumor genomic analyses in metastatic urachal carcinoma. Clinical Genitourinary Cancer. 2016;**14**(4):e449-e452. DOI: 10.1016/j.clgc.2016.03.013. Epub 2016 Mar 24

[19] Abrams J, Conley B, Mooney M, Zwiebel J, Chen A, Welch JJ, et al. National Cancer Institute's precision medicine initiatives for the new National Clinical Trials Network. American Society of Clinical Oncology Educational Book. 2014;**34**:71-76. DOI: 10.14694/EdBook_AM.2014.34.71

[20] Redig AJ, Jänne PA. Basket trials and the evolution of clinical trial design in an era of genomic medicine. Journal of Clinical Oncology. 2015;**33**(9):975-977. DOI: 10.1200/JCO.2014.59.8433. Epub 2015 Feb 9

[21] Kantor AF, Hartge P, Hoover RN, Fraumeni JF Jr. Epidemiological characteristics of squamous cell carcinoma and adenocarcinoma of the bladder. Cancer Research. 1988;**48**(13):3853-3855

[22] Fortuny J, Kogevinas M, Chang-Claude J, González CA, Hours M, Jöckel KH, et al. Tobacco, occupation and non-transitional-cell carcinoma of the bladder: An international case-control study. International Journal of Cancer. 1999;**80**(1):44-46. DOI: 10.1002/(sici)1097-0215(19990105)80:1<44::aid-ijc9>3.0.co;2-8

[23] Gordetsky JB, Montgomery KW, Giannico GA, Rais-Bahrami S, Thapa P, Boorjian S, et al. The significance of squamous histology on clinical outcomes and PD-L1 expression in bladder cancer. International Journal of Surgical Pathology. 2022;**30**(1):6-14. DOI: 10.1177/10668969211027264. Epub 2021 Jun 28

[24] Subramonian K, Cartwright RA, Harnden P, Harrison SC. Bladder cancer in patients with spinal cord injuries. BJU International. 2004;**93**(6):739-743. DOI: 10.1111/j.1464-410X.2003.04718.x

[25] Pannek J. Transitional cell carcinoma in patients with spinal cord injury: A high risk malignancy? Urology. 2002;**59**(2):240-244. DOI: 10.1016/s0090-4295(01)01495-9

[26] Hamid R, Bycroft J, Arya M, Shah PJ. Screening cystoscopy and biopsy in patients with neuropathic bladder and chronic suprapubic indwelling catheters: Is it valid? The Journal of Urology. 2003;**170**(2 Pt 1):425-427. DOI: 10.1097/01.ju.0000076700.00853.ad

[27] Yang CC, Clowers DE. Screening cystoscopy in chronically catheterized spinal cord injury patients. Spinal Cord. 1999;**37**(3):204-207. DOI: 10.1038/sj.sc.3100767

[28] Scosyrev E, Yao J, Messing E. Urothelial carcinoma versus squamous cell carcinoma of bladder: Is survival different with stage adjustment? Urology. 2009;**73**(4):822-827. DOI: 10.1016/j.urology.2008.11.042. Epub 2009 Feb 4

[29] Rundle JS, Hart AJ, McGeorge A, Smith JS, Malcolm AJ, Smith PM. Squamous cell carcinoma of bladder. A review of 114 patients. British Journal of Urology. 1982;**54**(5):522-526. DOI: 10.1111/j.1464-410x.1982.tb13580.x

[30] Swanson DA, Liles A, Zagars GK. Preoperative irradiation and radical cystectomy for stages T2 and T3 squamous cell carcinoma of the bladder. The Journal of Urology. 1990;**143**(1):37-40. DOI: 10.1016/s0022-5347(17)39857-9

[31] Richie JP, Waisman J, Skinner DG, Dretler SP. Squamous carcinoma of the bladder: Treatment by radical cystectomy. The Journal of Urology. 1976;**115**(6):670-672. DOI: 10.1016/s0022-5347(17)59330-1

[32] Tannenbaum SI, Carson CC 3rd, Tatum A, Paulson DF. Squamous carcinoma of urinary bladder. Urology. 1983;**22**(6):597-599. DOI: 10.1016/0090-4295(83)90303-5

[33] Baumann BC, Zaghloul MS, Sargos P, Murthy V. Adjuvant and neoadjuvant radiation therapy for locally advanced bladder cancer. Clinical Oncology (Royal College of Radiologists). 2021;**33**(6):391-399. DOI: 10.1016/j.clon.2021.03.020

[34] Fischer-Valuck BW, Michalski JM, Mitra N, Christodouleas JP, DeWees TA, Kim E, et al. Effectiveness of postoperative radiotherapy after radical cystectomy for locally advanced bladder cancer. Cancer Medicine. 2019;**8**(8):3698-3709. DOI: 10.1002/cam4.2102. Epub 2019 May 22

[35] Fischer-Valuck BW, Michalski JM, Harton JG, Birtle A, Christodouleas JP, Efstathiou JA, et al. Management of muscle-invasive bladder cancer during a pandemic: Impact of treatment delay on survival outcomes for patients treated with definitive concurrent chemoradiotherapy. Clinical Genitourinary Cancer. 2021;**19**(1):41-46.e1. DOI: 10.1016/j.clgc.2020.06.005. Epub 2020 Jun 22

[36] James ND, Hussain SA, Hall E, Jenkins P, Tremlett J, Rawlings C, et al. Radiotherapy with or without chemotherapy in muscle-invasive bladder cancer. The New England Journal of Medicine. 2012;**366**(16):1477-1488. DOI: 10.1056/NEJMoa1106106

[37] Flam M, John M, Pajak TF, Petrelli N, Myerson R, Doggett S, et al. Role of mitomycin in combination with fluorouracil and radiotherapy, and of salvage chemoradiation in the definitive nonsurgical treatment of epidermoid carcinoma of the anal canal: Results of a phase III randomized intergroup study. Journal of Clinical Oncology. 1996;**14**(9):2527-2539. DOI: 10.1200/JCO.1996.14.9.2527

[38] Ryan DP, Compton CC, Mayer RJ. Carcinoma of the anal canal. The New England Journal of Medicine. 2000;**342**(11):792-800. DOI: 10.1056/NEJM200003163421107

[39] Serretta V, Pomara G, Piazza F, Gange E. Pure squamous cell carcinoma of the bladder in western countries. Report on 19 consecutive cases. European Urology. 2000;**37**(1):85-89. DOI: 10.1159/000020105

[40] Galsky MD, Iasonos A, Mironov S, Scattergood J, Donat SM, Bochner BH, et al. Prospective trial of ifosfamide, paclitaxel, and cisplatin in patients with advanced non-transitional cell carcinoma of the urothelial tract. Urology. 2007;**69**(2):255-259. DOI: 10.1016/j.urology.2006.10.029

[41] Zahoor H, Elson P, Stephenson A, Haber GP, Kaouk J, Fergany A, et al. Patient characteristics, treatment patterns and prognostic factors in squamous cell bladder cancer. Clinical Genitourinary Cancer. 2018;**16**(2):e437-e442. DOI: 10.1016/j.clgc.2017.10.005. Epub 2017 Oct 17

[42] Rosenberg JE, Hoffman-Censits J, Powles T, van der Heijden MS, Balar AV, Necchi A, et al. Atezolizumab in patients with locally advanced and metastatic urothelial carcinoma who have progressed following treatment with platinum-based chemotherapy: A single-arm, multicentre, phase 2 trial. Lancet. 2016;**387**(10031):1909-1920. DOI: 10.1016/S0140-6736(16)00561-4. Epub 2016 Mar 4

[43] Bellmunt J, de Wit R, Vaughn DJ, Fradet Y, Lee JL, Fong L, et al. Pembrolizumab as second-line therapy for advanced urothelial carcinoma. The New England Journal of Medicine. 2017;**376**(11):1015-1026. DOI: 10.1056/NEJMoa1613683. Epub 2017 Feb 17

[44] Hussain M, Vaishampayan U, Du W, Redman B, Smith DC. Combination paclitaxel, carboplatin, and gemcitabine is an active treatment for advanced urothelial cancer. Journal of Clinical Oncology. 2001;**19**(9):2527-2533. DOI: 10.1200/JCO.2001.19.9.2527

[45] Nishiyama H, Habuchi T, Watanabe J, Teramukai S, Tada H, Ono Y, et al. Clinical outcome of a large-scale multi-institutional retrospective study for locally advanced bladder cancer: A survey including 1131 patients treated during 1990-2000 in Japan. European Urology. 2004;**45**(2):176-181. DOI: 10.1016/j.eururo.2003.09.011

Chapter 3

Epigenetic Regulation in Cancer and Cancer Therapies

Mehak Sharan, Runjhun Mathur, Niraj Kumar Jha, Khushboo Rana, Saurabh Kumar Jha and Abhimanyu Kumar Jha

Abstract

It has been believed that identification of alterations in epigenetic profiles can be used to distinguish not only between various types of malignancies but also between different phases of cancer progression. As a result, epigenetic factors have a lot of potential to become more accurate diagnostic and prognostic biomarkers for many malignancies. Although DNA methylation is the most researched aspect of epigenetics, only a few methylation markers are routinely used in clinical practice. DNA methylation biomarkers, on the other hand, are expected to play a significant role in the near future. To summarize, epigenetic regulation plays a critical role in cancer development, and epigenetic biomarker analysis has a lot of potential to become clinically useful. More research is needed to further develop and evaluate epigenetic biomarkers' therapeutic use.

Keywords: epigenetics, biomarkers, cancer, tumour suppressor genes, oncogenes, hypermethylation

1. Introduction

Cancer is a disease where some body's cells grow uncontrollably and spread to other parts of the body. The human cells can grow fast and multiply by cell division to forming new cells as the body required. When cells are growing old, damaged, or die, then new cells take their place. Sometimes the process of cycle breaks down, and abnormal or damaged cells can grow and multiply. This abnormal growth of cells may form tumours, which are lumps of tissue. Tumours can be divided into two types; cancerous or not cancerous (benign). Cancerous tumours spread into, or invade, nearby tissues which can travel to different places in the body to form new tumours by a process called metastasis. Cancerous tumours are called as malignant tumours. Sometimes benign tumours can also cause various serious symptoms in life; to be life-threatening, such as benign tumours in the brain. Cancer has long existed for all of human history [1]. In the earliest written history record, cancer has been circa 1600 BC in the Egyptian Edwin Smith Papyrus which is described as breast cancer [2].

In the fifteenth to seventeenth centuries, it became accepted by doctors to dissect bodies and discover the reason to cause of death [3]. According to German professor Wilhelm Fabry, it was believed that breast cancer was caused due to a milk clot in a mammary duct. His contemporary Nicolaes Tulp believed that it was a poison that can spreads slowly through outcome chemical process and acidic lymph fluid [4].

Cancer is a kind of disease which involves abnormal cell growth with lot of potential to invade or spread to other parts of the body [5, 6]. These contrast with benign tumours, which do not spread [7]. These symptoms including a lump, abnormal bleeding, prolonged cough, unexplained weight loss and a change in bowel movements [8].

Tobacco is one of the leading causes of cancer death, accounting for around 22% of all cancer fatalities [9]. Obesity, poor diet, lack of physical activity and excessive alcohol consumption account for another 10% of deaths [6–8]. Other concerns include diseases, ionizing radiation exposure and exposure to contaminants in the environment [10]. Helicobacter pylori, hepatitis B, hepatitis C, human papillomavirus infection, Epstein-Barr virus and human immunodeficiency virus (HIV) cause 15% of malignancies in the poor world [11]. Inherited genetic abnormalities are responsible for 5–10% of cancer cases [12].

No smoking, maintaining a healthy weight, limiting alcohol intake, eating plenty of vegetables, fruits and whole grains, vaccination against certain infectious diseases, limiting consumption of processed meat and red meat and limiting exposure to direct sunlight are all factors that can help prevent cancer [13, 14]. Cervical and colorectal cancers can be detected early by screening [15]. The benefits of breast cancer screening are debatable [15]. Radiation therapy, surgery, chemotherapy and targeted therapy are frequently used to treat cancer [5, 8]. In 15-year-old children who have been diagnosed with cancer, the 5-year survival rate for cancer in the industrialized world is on average 80%. The average 5-year survival rate in the United States is 66% [16].

About 8.8 million deaths were caused in 2019 (15.7% of deaths) [17]. The most common types of cancer in males are lung cancer, prostate cancer, colorectal cancer and stomach cancer [18]. In females, the most common types are breast cancer, colorectal cancer, lung cancer and cervical cancer [19].

2. Causes of cancer

Genetic alterations generated by environmental and lifestyle factors cause 90–95% of cancer cases [8]. Inherited genetics is responsible for the remaining 5–10% [8]. Environmental influences include, lifestyle, economic and behavioural factors, as well as pollution, but they are not inherited. Tobacco use (25–30%), food and obesity (30–35%), infections (15–20%), radiation (both ionizing and non-ionizing, up to 10%), lack of physical activity and pollution are all common environmental factors that can contribute to cancer death [8, 19]. Psychological stress does not appear to be a risk factor for cancer start [19, 20], but it may affect outcomes in people who have already been diagnosed with cancer [20].

3. Epidemiology

The cancer epidemiology provides the various types of essential information on causes and population trends of these conditions. It is possible to establish timely and appropriate healthcare interventions aimed at developing efficient policies for prevention, screening and diagnosis [1]. Recently, a concise overview on current cancer epidemiologic data is described which was gathered from the official databases of the World Health Organization (WHO) and American Cancer Society (ACS) in an attempt of providing updated information on frequency, mortality and survival expectancy of the 15 leading types of cancers worldwide. According to estimates, there were 18.1 million new cancer diagnoses and 9.6 million deaths worldwide in 2018 [20] as shown in **Figure 1**. About 20% of males and 17% of females will develop cancer at some point in their lives, with 13% of males and 9% of females dying from it [20].

In 2008, around 12.7 million malignancies (excluding non-melanoma skin cancers) were diagnosed, and nearly 7.98 million people died [18]. Cancer is responsible for about 16% of all fatalities. Lung cancer (1.76 million deaths in 2018), colorectal cancer (860,000), stomach cancer (780,000), liver cancer (780,000) and breast cancer (620,000) are the most common [5]. Invasive cancer is thus the major cause of death in developed countries and the second leading cause in developing countries [19]. The developing world accounts for more than half of all cases [20].

In 1990, 5.8 million people died of cancer [18]. Longer life spans and lifestyle changes in the developing countries have contributed to an increase in deaths [18]. Age is the single most important risk factor for cancer [19]. Although cancer can strike at any age, the majority of people with aggressive cancer are over 65 [20].

Aging's effect on cancer is complicated by factors such as DNA damage and inflammation promoting it and factors such as vascular aging and endocrine changes inhibiting it [20].

Leukaemia (34%), brain tumours (23%) and lymphomas (12%) are the three most prevalent childhood cancers [20]. In the United States, one out of every 285 children is diagnosed with cancer. Childhood cancer rates grew by 0.6% per year in the United States between 1975 and 2002 and by 1.1% per year in Europe between 1978 and 1997 [20].

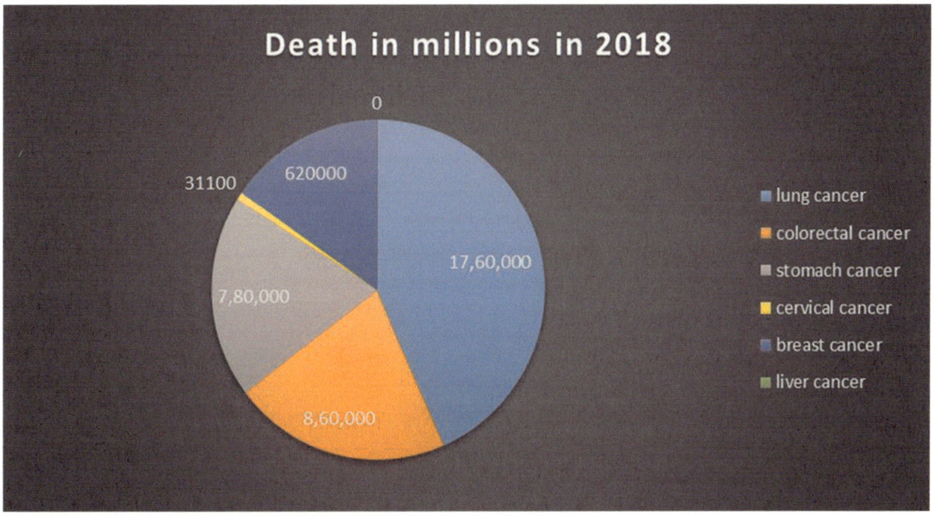

Figure 1.
Estimates of deaths due to cancer in 2018.

4. Types of cancer

A total of 100 cancer kinds have been found. Cancers are frequently called after the organs or tissues in which they develop. Lung cancer, for example, begins in the lungs, while brain cancer begins in the brain. Cancers can also be classified based on the type of cell that caused them, such as epithelial or squamous cells. Most cancers are named for the organ or type of cell in which they start—for example, cancer that begins in the colon is called colon cancer; cancer that begins in melanocytes of the skin is called melanoma. The following includes a description of the major cancer types.

4.1 Brain and central nervous system cancer

Cancers of the brain and central nervous system (CNS) are abnormal cell growths in the brain and spinal cord tissues. Primary brain tumours are cancers that start in the brain. A metastatic brain tumour is a tumour that begins in another part of the body and travels to the brain.

It may be either benign (not cancer) or malignant (cancer). The symptoms of brain and spinal cord tumours depend on where the tumour forms, its size, how fast it is growing and the age of the patient. In adults, anaplastic astrocytomas and glioblastomas make up about one-third of brain tumours. In children, astrocytomas are the most common type of brain tumour. Seizures, drowsiness, confusion and behavioural abnormalities are only some of the signs of brain cancer. Although the causes of brain tumours are unknown, several risk factors include hereditary or genetic disorders, as well as exposure to extremely high doses of radiation to the head. Surgery, radiation, chemotherapy or steroid therapy, or a combination of these treatments, may be used to treat brain tumours [20, 21].

4.2 Breast cancer

Breast cancer is a disease in which the cells of the breast grow out of control. It only affects women. Ductal carcinoma is the most prevalent type of breast cancer, which begins in the cells of the ducts. Breast cancer develops in the cells of the lobules and other breast tissues. Breast cancer spreads to surrounding tissue from where it begins in the ducts or lobules. Many forms of breast cancer can develop a lump in the breast, but not all of them do. New lumps or thickening in the breast or under the arm, nipple discharge or turning in, nipple ulcers, skin of the breast dimpling and rash or red swollen breasts are some of the signs and symptoms. The causes of breast cancer are unknown, but risk factors include increasing age, family history, inheritance of mutations, exposure to female hormones (natural and administered), obesity (poor diet and inadequate exercise) and excess alcohol consumption [22, 23].

4.3 Cervical cancer

Cervical cancer happens when abnormal cells on the cervix, the lower part of the uterus (womb), grow out of control. Squamous cell carcinoma (which accounts for 80% of cases) and adenocarcinoma are two types of cervical cancer. The thin, flat cells that border the cervix are where squamous cell cancer develops. Cervical cells that produce mucus and other fluids are where adenocarcinoma originates. Because it begins higher in the cervix, adenocarcinoma is less prevalent and more difficult to identify. Cervical cell alterations that occur early on rarely cause symptoms. Vaginal bleeding in between periods, menstrual bleeding that is longer or heavier than usual, bleeding after intercourse, pain during intercourse, unusual vaginal discharge, vaginal bleeding after menopause, excessive tiredness, leg pain or swelling and low back pain are some of the most common symptoms. Almost all occurrences of cervical cancer are caused by long-term infections with certain forms of human papillomavirus. The other major cause of cervical cancer is smoking. Cervical cancer can be squamous cell carcinoma (accounting for 80% of cases) and adenocarcinoma. Squamous cell carcinoma begins in the thin, flat cells that line the cervix. Adenocarcinoma begins in cervical cells that make mucus and other fluids. Adenocarcinoma is less common and more difficult to diagnose because it starts higher in the cervix. Early changes in cervical cells rarely cause symptoms. The most common signs are vaginal bleeding between periods, menstrual bleeding may be longer or heavier than usual, bleeding after intercourse, pain during intercourse, unusual vaginal discharge, vaginal bleeding after menopause, excessive tiredness, leg pain or swelling and low back pain. Long-lasting infections with certain types of human papillomavirus cause almost all cases of cervical cancer. The other main risk factor for cervical cancer is smoking. Treatment may include surgery, radiation therapy, chemotherapy or a combination. The choice of treatment depends on the size of the tumour and disease stage [24, 25].

4.4 Oesophageal cancer

Oesophageal cancer forms in the tissues of the oesophagus. The most common types of oesophageal cancer are squamous cell carcinoma and adenocarcinoma. The upper and middle oesophagus are the most common sites for this malignancy; however, it can arise anywhere throughout the oesophagus. Epidermoid carcinoma is another name for this condition. Adenocarcinoma is a cancer that starts in glandular (secretory) cells, which produce and leak mucus and other fluids. It normally develops near the stomach in the lower section of the oesophagus. Oesophageal cancer is increased by smoking, heavy alcohol consumption and Barrett oesophagus. Barrett oesophagus and gastroesophageal reflux disease may raise the risk of oesophageal cancer. Weight loss, hoarseness and cough and painful or difficult swallowing are all signs and symptoms of oesophageal cancer. Because there are no early indications or symptoms, oesophageal cancer is frequently identified at an advanced stage. Doctors frequently prescribe combining multiple types of treatment for persons with tumours that have not migrated beyond the oesophagus and lymph nodes, such as radiation therapy, chemotherapy and surgery. The order in which therapies are given varies depending on a number of criteria, including the type of oesophageal cancer [26, 27].

4.5 Head and neck cancer

About 90% cases of cancers found in head and neck begin in the squamous cells that line the moist, mucosal surfaces inside the head and neck and are known as head and neck squamous cell carcinoma (HNSCC). HNSCC is the sixth leading cancer by incidence worldwide. The tumour, node, metastasis (TNM) staging system may be often used to classify patients with HNSCC and also based on the clinical, radiological and pathological examination of tumour specimens [28]. Head and neck cancer area may become metastatic and spread to several types of organs or tissues such as the brain and lung through lymphatic and blood vessels. Amplification of region 11q13, 7p11 and other chromosomal aberrations have also been linked to HNSCC progression [29]. Tobacco usage and alcohol use are two of the most dangerous risk factors associated to this malignancy: a lump or sore that does not heal, a persistent sore throat, difficulty swallowing, a change or hoarseness in the voice and other symptoms [30]. Patients with HNSCC have a 5-year survival rate of approximately 40%–50%. If discovered and treated early, head and neck cancer is highly curable [31]. Chromosomal abnormalities such as amplification of region 11q13, 7p11, etc. are also associated with HNSCC aggravation [29]. There are several risk factors linked to this cancer, the most vicious ones are tobacco use and alcohol consumption. Symptoms may include a lump or sore that does not heal, a sore throat that does not go away, trouble in swallowing, a change or hoarseness in the voice, etc. [30]. The 5-year survival rate of patients with HNSCC is about 40%–50%. Head and neck cancer is highly curable if detected and treated early [31]. Head and neck cancer can be managed either in prophylactic manner, i.e. stoppage of alcohol consumption and smoking habit, grinding of sharp cuspal teeth, ultrasonic scaling, etc. or through definitive management such as surgical removal, chemotherapy, etc.

4.6 Liver cancer

Liver cancer is called as hepatic cancer or hepatocellular carcinoma. It starts from the tissue of the liver. In other words, it is a primary liver cancer. Cancer is spread from elsewhere to the liver, known as liver metastasis which is more common than primary liver cancer. Liver cancer is rare in children and teenagers, but there are two types of liver cancer that can form in children Cholangiocarcinoma is another name for bile duct cancer. Intrahepatic cholangiocarcinoma is a type of cancer that begins in the bile ducts of the liver. Extrahepatic cholangiocarcinoma is a type of cholangiocarcinoma that begins in the bile ducts outside of the liver. Compared with intrahepatic cholangiocarcinoma, extrahepatic cholangiocarcinoma is substantially more prevalent.

The signs and symptoms of liver cancer are often not felt or detected until the illness has progressed significantly. Unintentional weight loss, loss of appetite, feeling very full after eating, even if the meal was modest, feeling ill and vomiting, pain or swelling in your abdomen (tummy), jaundice and itchy skin are some of the symptoms that might occur [32–34].

4.7 Leukaemia

Leukaemia is a hematopoietic stem cell–initiated heterogeneous disease which occurs in abnormal blood cell proliferation in the bone marrow and peripheral blood [35]. It can affect very fast (lymphocytes or myelocytes). The four main types of leukaemia may include chronic lymphocytic leukaemia (CLL), acute lymphocytic leukaemia, acute myelocytic leukaemia and chronic myelocytic leukaemia. Leukaemia is usually present in white blood cells. However, red blood cells and platelets may also become cancerous. Pain in the bones or joints, swollen lymph nodes that do not really hurt, fever or night sweats, feeling weak or weary, bleeding and bruising easily, frequent infections, discomfort or swelling in the belly, weight loss or loss of appetite are all common symptoms of chronic or acute leukaemia. Chemotherapy is used to treat the majority of leukaemia patients. Radiation therapy /or bone marrow transplantation may be used in some patients [36, 37].

4.8 Lung cancer

Lung cancer is a form of cancer that starts in the trachea (windpipe), bronchus (main airway) or lung tissue. Non-small-cell lung cancer and small-cell lung cancer are the two most common kinds of lung cancer. Squamous cell carcinoma, adenocarcinoma and large cell carcinoma are all subtypes of non-small-cell lung cancer. Small cell lung cancer is also called oat cell cancer. About 10%–15% of lung cancers are small-cell lung cancers. Cigarette smoking is the principal risk factor for development of lung cancer, but many people with the condition eventually develop symptoms including a persistent cough, coughing up blood, persistent breathlessness, unexplained tiredness and weight loss and an ache or pain when breathing or coughing. Treatment of lung cancer can involve a combination of surgery, chemotherapy and radiation therapy as well as newer experimental methods

4.9 Pancreatic cancer

Pancreatic cancer is caused due to abnormal and uncontrolled growth of cells in the pancreas—a large gland that is part of the digestive system. Adenocarcinomas are most commonly found in gland cells in the pancreatic ducts, although they can also occur in pancreatic enzyme cells (acinar cell carcinoma). Adenosquamous carcinomas, squamous cell carcinomas and giant cell carcinomas, all named by their appearances under a microscope, are further types of pancreatic tumours linked to exocrine activities. For example, insulinomas (insulin), glucagonomas (glucagon), gastrinomas (gastrin), somatostatinomas (somatostatin) and VIPomas (vasoactive intestinal peptide or VIP). Functioning islet cell tumours still make hormones, while nonfunctioning ones do not. Symptoms may include abdominal pain, weight loss, diarrhoea and jaundice. They can also be caused by conditions such as pancreatitis (inflammation of the pancreas), gallstones, irritable bowel syndrome or hepatitis (inflammation of the liver). Smoking is one of the most important risk factors for pancreatic cancer. Heavy exposure at work to certain chemicals used in the dry cleaning and metal working industries may raise a person's risk of pancreatic cancer. Surgery, radiation and chemotherapy are the most common treatment types.

4.10 Prostate cancer

Men are the only ones who get prostate cancer. The prostate gland, which is part of the male reproductive system, is where cancer starts to grow. Localized prostate cancer, also known as early prostate cancer, is cancer that is contained within the prostate and does not cause any symptoms. Adenocarcinomas are the most common type of prostate cancer (cancers that begin in cells that make and release mucus and other fluids). Early indications of prostate cancer are frequently absent. Men with advanced prostate cancer may have more frequent urination or a weaker urine flow, although these symptoms can also be caused by benign prostate diseases. The following symptoms may occur if a tumour causes the prostate gland to enlarge or if cancer spreads beyond the prostate: Frequent urination, a painful or burning sensation during urination or ejaculation, blood in urine or sperm and pain or stiffness in the lower back, hips, pelvis or thighs are all symptoms of urinary incontinence. In fact, males over the age of 65 account for more than 65% of all prostate cancer diagnoses.

Various other cancers are bladder cancer, colorectal cancer, gastric cancer, sarcoma, kidney cancer, lymphoma, melanoma, ovarian cancer (**Table 1**).

Cancer	Affected body part
Brain and central nervous system cancer	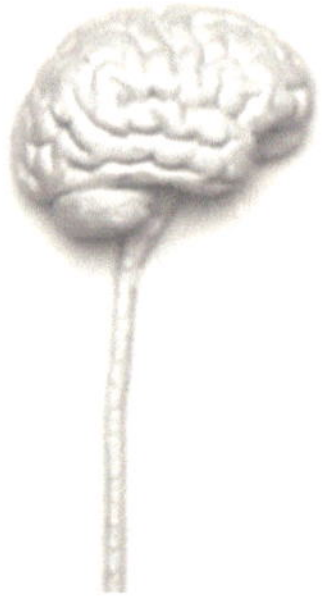
Breast cancer	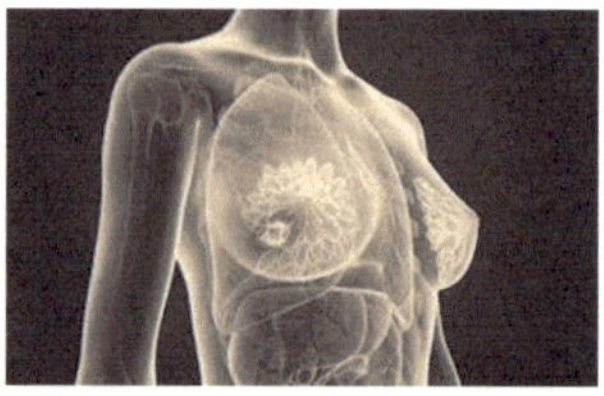
Cervical cancer	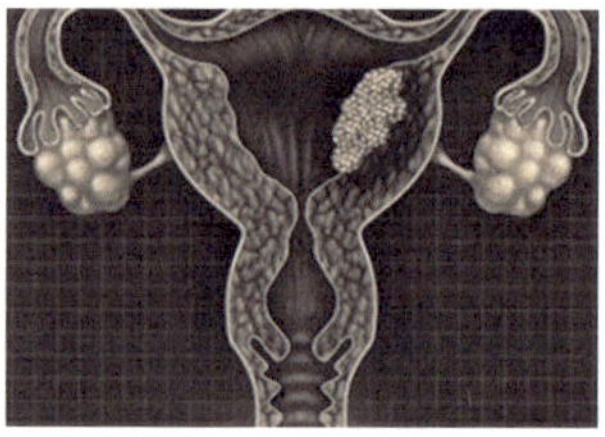
Oesophageal cancer	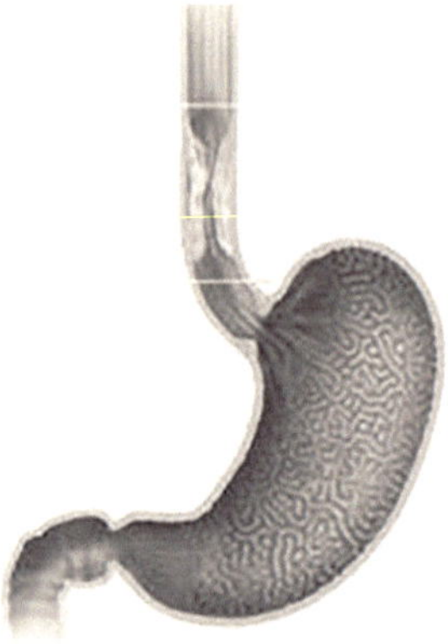
Head and neck cancer	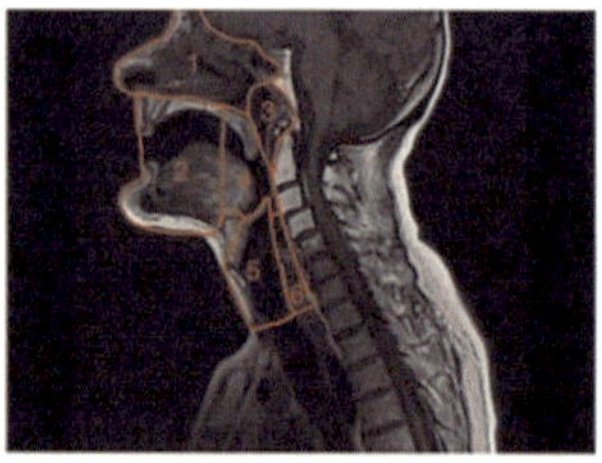

Cancer	Affected body part
Liver cancer	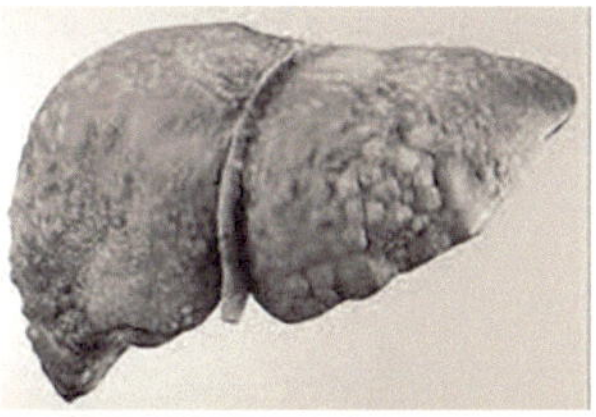
Leukaemia	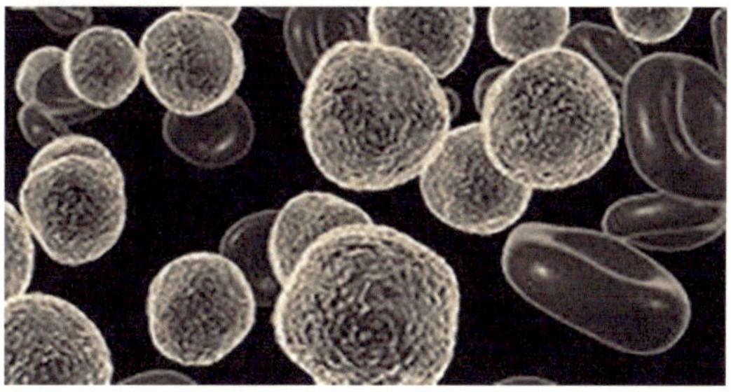
Lung cancer	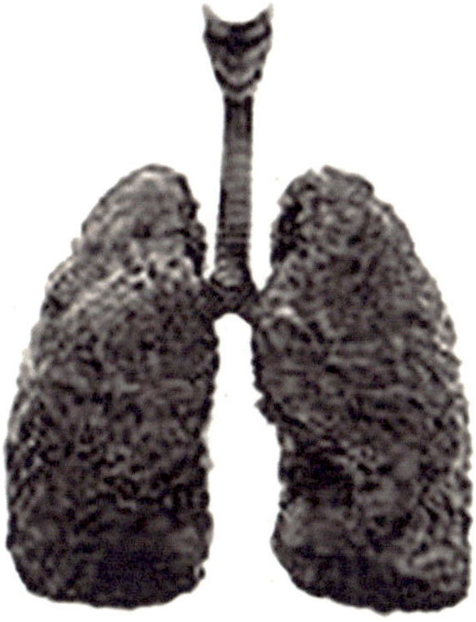
Pancreatic cancer	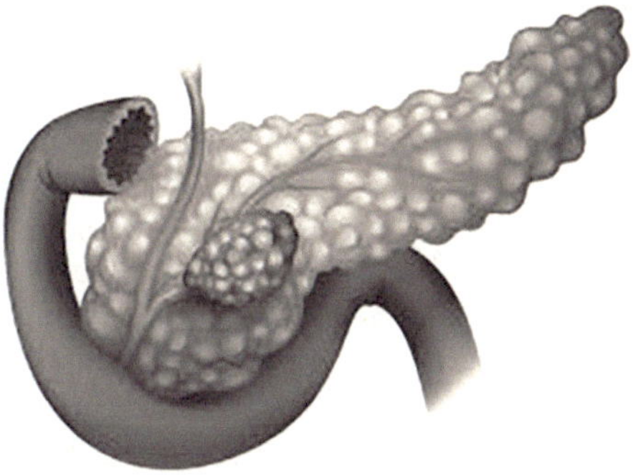

Cancer	Affected body part
Prostate cancer	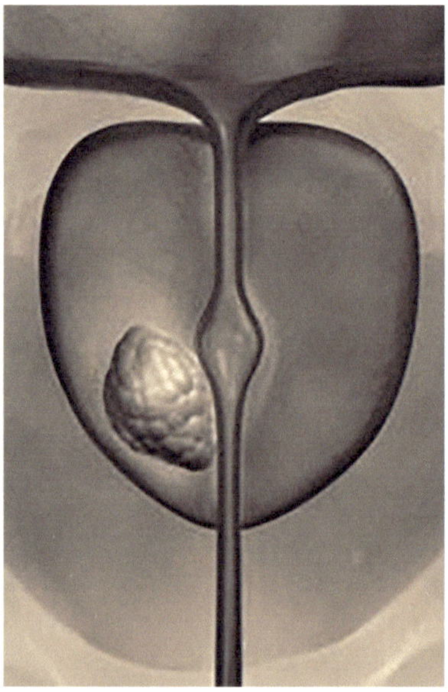

Table 1.
Types of cancer and body parts it affects.

5. Epigenetic factors

The abnormal patterns such as the change in composition of chromatin or organization of chromatin, DNA methylation, disrupted patterns in the post translational modifications of histone are known as the epigenetic alterations. These changes in the epigenomes might occur by the disruption on the epigenetic machinery which are associated with the mutated patterns of the wild-type genes expressions along with their changed states. In the process of tumorigenesis, the epigenetic component recognition is important for a better understanding of the cancer along with new research in treatment, detection and prevention of cancer. The mutations in oncogene or the signalling gene in any human cancer are dominant that lead to formation of tumours and cancer. For an instance, the activity of the product of gene for growth stimulation is enhanced due to the mutation in the gene, ras. These types of epigenetic silencing of tumour suppressor genes or the genetic mutations in these genes are often observed to be recessive that requires the disruption in both the copies of alleles in order to get the full expression of the phenotype which is transformed.

Two or multiple-hit hypothesis: According to the study of Knudson [38] in 2001, the hypothesis of the two or multiple hit was proposed as the idea that in the malignant cell line, the two copies of tumour suppressor genes have to be incapacitated. The three classes' hits can work in combinations of different types in order to cause the complete loss of activity of tumour suppressor genes. The mutations in the coding sequence along with loss of either entire copies or part of copies of genes, the silencing of epigenetics might occur to cooperate to lead to disable the control of gene.

There are studies that signify that the cancers harbour the mutations that are frequent in genes for the epigenetic machinery that lead to abnormalities in epigenome. These abnormalities affect the gene patterns of expressions along with the stability [39]. There are genes that are frequently mutated, especially the ones that encode proteins responsible for the normal chromatin control of the DNA methylation [40]. These patterns are important to understand the cancer biology along with the new discoveries in the cancer therapy. The epigenetic activation or silencing of genes may lead to cells for mutations such as the epigenetic silencing of the MLH1 DNA repair protein as it leads to lack of efficient DNA repair. There are epigenetics processed that regulate the genome and could be downregulated in cancer.

Whole exon sequencing, genome-wide DNA methylation, RNA expression, whole genome sequencing and chromatin analyses' results showed the understanding of the epigenomes in the normal and cancer cells [41]. This signified that the epigenetic control not only comprises the coding genes but also the microRNAs, non-coding RNAs and other genome regulatory functions [42]. These mutations are present in high frequencies and known as the 'driver' mutations that result in the disruption of the epigenome by mutations for the invasion and progression of cancer. These epigenetic changes take place independently of the mutations in factors of chromatin modification where the damage and heritable alterations are induced due to the physiological or environmental events in cancer progression or inheritance of cancer risk states [43].

The very first proposal of the alteration in DNA methylation as a contribution to cancer was the discovery of the methylation of the cytosine in DNA to become 5-methylcytosine. There have been many studies on 5mC alterations and its distribution pattern that can help to distinguish it from the normal cells with the result of three major routes. The three major routes involved in the CpG methylation in the oncogenic phenotype are by: hypomethylation on oncogenes, hypermethylation of tumour suppressor genes and mutagenesis of 5mC by UV radiation, carcinogens or deamination [44].

6. Hypomethylation of oncogenes

The DNA methylation changes in cancer cells with regional modifications which is recognized as the global DNA hypomethylation by the genome-wide analyses [45]. The genomic instability with increase in aneuploidy is the result of the DNA demethylation that could act as a hallmark of cancer. The reduction and deletion of DNA methyltransferase, DNMT1 could result in the tumour induction along with increased mutation and aneuploidies rates. It clearly indicates the chromosomal fragility [46]. The activation of transcription by transcription of oncogenes, repeats and transposable elements is accompanied by the loss of DNA methylation [45]. The activation of the transposable elements acts as source of potential mutations during the process of transposition. The genome has CpG islands which are around 80% methylated, and in cancer this methylation rate drops to 40–60%. The mapping technologies available could be useful in detecting the patterns more precisely. About one-third of the genome could be covered with the blocks of DNA hypomethylated blocks of 28kb–10Mb. The cause of this is hypothesized by many theories such as the DNA hypomethylation could be associated with broad shifts in chromatin organization that could result in mutations affecting the homeostasis of DNA methylation.

7. Direct mutagenesis

The methylation of the cytosine in somatic cells is more than one-third of all the transitional mutations observed. The somatic mutations in the cancer-causing p53 gene were studied (Rideout et al. 1990). This mechanism is common in somatic tissues and forms many inactivating mutations in tumour suppressor genes due to the methylation of the fifth position of cytosine ring that in the double-standard DNA increases the hydrolytic deamination. The product of deamination of 5mC is thymine and not uracil, and so the DNA repair mechanism is less efficient to repair this mismatch. For example, among all the p53 mutations, more than 50% of the mutations or methylation occurs in the cytosine area [47]. Thus, the risk of the cancer increases by the endogenous mechanism. The cytosine methylation favours the carcinogenic adducts between the carcinogens and DNA like the cigarette smoke that result in the increased mutation sites in the CpG sites of lungs [47]. This type of direct mutagenesis and DNA methylation can also alter the rate of mutations by factors such as sunlight-exposed skin as the methyl group changes the absorption spectrum for cytosine into normal incident sunlight [47].

8. Hypermethylation of TSG

The abnormal hypermethylation of the CpG islands in the five regions of cancer-related genes is associated with the transcriptional silencing along with the alternative mechanism to inactivate the tumour suppressor genes by mutation [48]. In normal development or the cell renewal systems, around 60% of all the gene promoters have then non-methylated CpG islands. This non-methylation of the chromatin is either active or ready to be activated to express the genes. The prevalence of the methylated CpG island promoters in the cancer cells is more that leads to conclusion that they are directly involved in the carcinogenesis. This could lead to new era of cancer therapy by the reversal of the epigenetic changes observed in cancer [49]. The methylation of the gene body gives rise to elongation during transcription and enhancing the gene expression; thus, 5mC is more common in gene body of active genes and is associated with this rather than repression [50].

9. Aberrant hypermethylation

The loss of function of gene acts as a mediator between the abnormalities caused by epigenetic and genetic changes. There is always a debate over the cause of cancer to be genetic or epigenetic. Although the combination of these two factors works towards the tumour progression. The chromatin changes that lead to the gene function changes are important to understand the cancer mechanism and to develop the early detection and profiling of tumour with new targets for its prevention.

The silencing of genes that are important for transcription as they are associated with methylation of DNA in promoter regions of unmethylated gene [51, 52]. The increased emphasis on the delineation of the genes with new screening approaches now holds the important feature in research [53, 54]. In human cancers, there are number of genes that are hypermethylated which are mutated in the germline [1]. The common examples of hypermethylated genes are BRCA-1, MLH1, VHL, APC, E-cadherin, Rb, LKB1 and p16. They exhibit the non-familial cancers changes along with selective advantage in several ways for the loss of function of gene [55].

There are three types of characteristics of the aberrant hypermethylation: There are genes where the hypermethylation is observed in the specific tumour types. Secondly, there are genes that predict the phenotype of the tumour by the loss of specific function by epigenetic and genetic changes. Thirdly, there could be disruption in the pathways of the cells. There are several hyperemethylated genes, and in some of the genes, the methylation of the promoter is the only type of inactivation detected in the cancer as other genes are either rare or not have been observed. Each of the genes that are detected as hypermethylated must be identified and studied for its role in tumour type and progression. This is crucial as according to some studies, the genes that are hypermethylated could be mutated in a group and be responsible for the change in process or processes in biology of cancer such as in the repair of mismatch mutation [56, 57]. The non-critical and critical loci are affected by both the processes, leading to tumour development by loss of function of the key gene.

The CpG islands that are hypermethylated have been identified as a guide to clone the tumour suppressor genes that are frequently observed to be deleted in several cancers, but no genetic alterations have been identified in the tumour suppressor genes [58]. For example, the member of the zinc-finger transcription factor family, HIC-1, showed its importance in the process of development in hypermethylation in many tumours [59, 60] and also upregulated by the protein, p53 [10, 13]. The role of the gene is still under study, but the death of mice during embryogenesis from various defects has been observed during the knock-out of HIC-1 [61]. This information obtained is very helpful because of the databases built up for the chromosome positions where the gene is located and helps in screening of the hypermethylated loci in the DNA of the tumour cells.

Hypermethylation is the early event in the progression of tumour, and when the hypermethylated promoter region increases in the normal cells and tissues, that mark the early stage. In tumorigenesis, the promoter hypermethylation of genes plays a vital role that could be detected in the early stages. The early losses of the control of the cell cycle, disruption of cell-to-cell signalling, altered transcription factors and genetic instability are the early genetic alterations to characterize human cancer. Loss of function of p16 gene by the epigenetic loss helps to pass the check points of the mortality to enter in onset of cellular immortality in carcinogenesis [62, 63] along with tumours in early stage [64, 65]. In colon cancer, the gatekeeper gene, APC, which is responsible for the transcription pathway of beta-catenin-TCF transcriptional pathway, gets hypermethylated, leading to onset of colon cancer [66]. Similarly, in breast cancer, the hypermethylation of E-cadherin promoter disrupts the cell-to-cell recognition that is observed in the early stages [67].

There are some basic differences between the promoter hypermethylation caused by genetic and epigenetic factors. Firstly, the loss of gene function with promoter hypermethylation is relatively more subtle selective than mutation in the tumour progression. As in genetic events, both alleles are disrupted in two-hit paradigm for loss of gene function of tumour suppressor gene. In this, the first genetic hits result in the haplo insufficiency states [68]. On the contrary, the loss of the gene transcription is related to aberrant hypermethylation of CpG island, which is mediated by the region-oriented methylation density [69]. This density can increase over time by the cell replication which is associated with the increase in transcription loss [70]. Secondly, the aberrant hypermethylation and gene silencing are potentially reversible even after being very stable in cancer cells, but the mutations on genetic level are not [71]. Most of the cells in epithelial tumours can form metastatic foci and could be highly invasive and can help in the invasion of tumour cells. This invasion requires re-expression of E-cadherin so that cell aggregates are formed by tumour cells to survive in the foreign environment [72]. This heterogeneous loss of E-cadherin in tumour sites of both primary and metastic phases in same patient is similar [73, 74]. Loss of function of E-cadherin is very common in epithelial cancers and mainly related to the promoter hypermethylation as the heaviest promoter hypermethylation occurs in most highly invasice cells [37]. Thus, the reversibility of the aberrant hypermethylation plays a key role in the dynamic of the cell population to detect the behaviour of tumour. The chromatin formation dynamics in the DNA methylation along with the deacetylation of histone works in tumours to silence the hypermethylated genes. There are certain hypermethylated genes that do no re-express even by the agents such as Trichostatin. This drug is although effective for minimal de-methylation. 5-aza-cytidine is the demethylating drug that could be used to achieve demthylation even in the low doses [75].

10. Tumour suppressor genes

During interaction between cells with its surroundings and cell proliferation, there are specific controls at every step, but alterations in them lead to tumour formation and its metastasis. This causes disturbance in the relation between the number of cells increment during cell division or decrease in number of cells due to apoptosis or differentiation. There are positive and negative signals that control the cell multiplication and the homeostasis maintenance, their effects are based on the genetic changes that affect the control points due to the tumorigenicity [76]. The malignancy is due to the genetic changes and control points which is now possible to identify and characterize. There are several changes detected in genes that led to tumour formation, and these alterations may have positive influence or can involve in inhibition of cell growth [77]. Tumorigenesis is a multi-step process that requires the different genetic changes with proper mechanism to be interpreted from the epidemiological studies. The altered cells population may increase due to the expansion of genetic change that leads to larger target pool of subsequent genetic changes. These alterations are mainly deletions and point mutations that lead to loss of function of genes that interfere with the process of restraining cell multiplication, leading to oncogenesis. This genetic alteration could give positive signals such as gene overexpression that could lead to gene amplification in signal transduction element that acts as a stimulus to cell proliferation.

There are different terms that are being used for these altered genes such as anti-oncogenes, tumour suppressor genes or recessive oncogenes. The terminology of these genes still does not satisfy the mechanism of their work as their existence to only inhibit action of oncogenes is not confirmed. Although there are genes that inhibit the proliferation and expression of proto-oncogenes. The negative influence of these genes has been confirmed by the neoplastic transformation, loss of heterozygosity in tumours and familial cancer. Loss of function of the normal alleles leading to the neoplastic transformation is the primary evidence by somatic cell hybrid experiment of genetic alterations. When injected into the host without loss of chromosome, none of the hybrids that were generated between tumorigenic and non-tumorigenic cells gave rise to tumours [78]. Thus, the rise of tumours from tumorigenic hybrid cells was confirmed by the specific chromosome losses which is usually suppressed in the normal cells. This phenomenon was achieved by the wide variety of tumour suppressor genes that were suppressed by the mutations or genetic alterations which lead to recessive genetic changes, complemented by the normal alleles from normal parents. There have been cases where the combinations of the tumour cell lines and non-tumorigenic cell line both showed the recessive changes that signified the presence of multiple alterations or combination of it [79]. There are several tumour suppressor genes reported for different cancers.

11. P53

TP53 is the gene that is responsible for the protein p53. This a gene is known as the guardian of the genome or the caretaker gene. This protein serves different functions in the cell such as regulation of cell cycle, DNA repair, transcription and apoptosis induction. When this tumour suppressor gene gets mutated, that leads to cause many cancers. It comprises 37% of the cancers reported in the world with 6.5 million diagnosed cases. The homozygous loss of this gene leads cancers with percentage of 65% in colon cancers, 50% in lung cancer and 30–50% in the breast cancers [80]. In leukaemia, sarcomas, lymphomas and neurogenic tumours, loss of p53 is also reported.

12. pRB

The first tumour suppressor protein that was discovered was pRB in the human retinoblastoma. It is a tumour survival factor that acts as a gatekeeper gene that functions in the cell division and death regulation and cell proliferation [81]. If mutation occurs in this gene, then the function is lost, and there is no control in the cell division leading to unlimited growth.

13. BCL2

The family of proteins either inhibits or induces cell apoptosis along with maintaining the mitochondria composition. The signalling cascade from mitochondria till the cell apoptosis is performed due to this gene [82].

These are the epigenetic factors that are involved in the regulation of cancer. There are many studies conducted to discover the epigenetic regulation in many cancers. One of the cancers with 54.5% mortality rate (WHO, 2018) is cervical cancer. There are many epigenetic regulations studied under it.

14. Epigenetic regulation in cervical cancer

DNA methylation and histone acetylation are the two most widely studied epigenetic factors. Although there are certain different factors such as RNA interference that could be responsible for the transcriptional silencing [83]. The main epigenetic alterations involved in the cervical cancer are illustrated in **Figure 2**.

Hypermethylated and hypomethylated genes: In the development of cervical cancer, infection by high risk type Human Papillomavirus (HPV) is one of the main causes. HPV 16 and HPV 18 are the two most known viruses to cause cervical cancer. In the genome of HPV, there are certain epigenetic changes that could be responsible for the carcinogenic process driven by the virus along with the genome of the host. The methylation machinery activation is one of the defence mechanisms adopted by the host during infection, when the viral gene is inserted into the host genome [84].

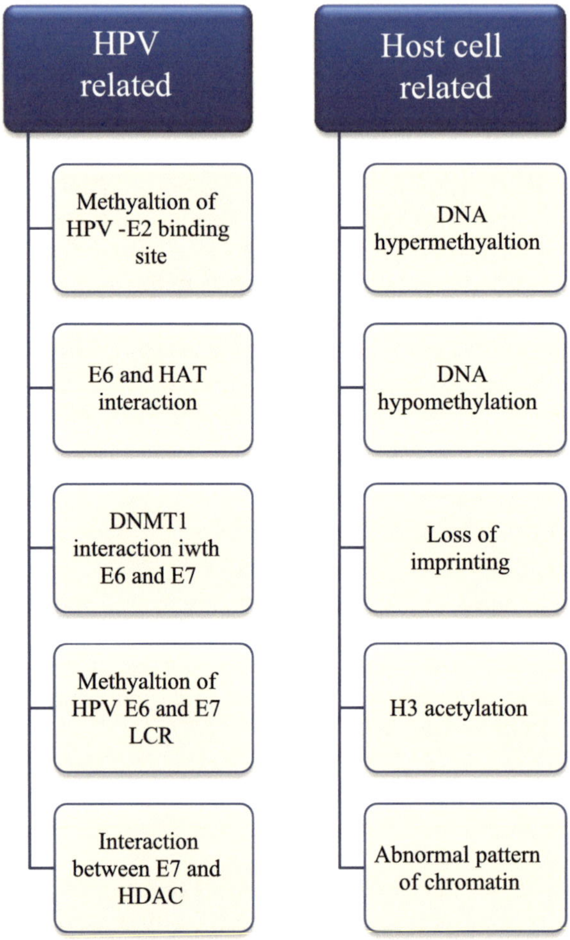

Figure 2.
Epigenetic alterations involved in the cervical cancer.

The activation of the silenced sequences in the human genomic DNA sequence with long terminal repeats and transposable elements could play a role in the process of cancer [85]. Viruses have the ability to regulate the expression of genes by methylation them in order to silence their activity to favour the infection [85]. On the other hand, viral genome can also synthesize oncoproteins that could either indirectly or directly silence the genes that may act against the tumour promotion. In a study of transfection of cell having methylated genome with HPV-16, it was observed that the DNA was transcriptionally repressed [86]. SiHa and CasKi are the two forms of cervical cancer cell lines that harbour the HPV-16 infection and have multiple viral genome copies. In one of the cases, it was found by the help of McfBC enzyme that the both cell lines when infected with HPV-16 have a conserved CpG hypo and hypermethylated genes. Hypermethylation of genes was found in 52% of the smears from asymptomatic women, 21.7% in pre-invasive lesions and 6.1% invasive case smears. Hypomethylation of LCR and E6 gene region of the oncogene was also observed. On the contrary to the first case study, high methylation frequency at most sites in carcinomas was found as compared with dysplasia and chromosomal integration in invasive lesions [87]. HPV 18 study was also studied in the two cervical cell lines, HeLa and C4-1. A clonal heterogeneity in the status of methylation was reported along with promoter methylation in 50% cancers and 66% smears. This resulted in the conclusion that the viral oncogenes in lesions are the result of their activity level in transcription and not neoplastic progression.

In HPV life cycle, E2 gene plays a key role in multiple processes such as viral DNA replication and transcription. A methylation analysis study on the E2-binding site within LCR on epithelial cervical cancer cell line from HPV-16-infected patient was done, and it was demonstrated that poorly differentiated basal cells were hypermethylated and that particular region of E2-binding site was hypomethylated [88]. Thus, the change of methylation status of viral genome during its life cycle could be helpful in detecting a novel means to modulate functioning of E2 to inhibit its progression.

Apoptosis-related genes: The study of these types of genes being affected by the methylation in cervical cancer is very less. The decoy receptors, DcR1 and DcR2, could serve as the easy target for the abnormal methylation that could lead to their silencing and losing their function [89]. DcR genes are the members of Tumour Necrosis Factors (TNFs) which include, Fas, TNFR1 and decoy receptors for TRAIL. DcR1 and DcR2 are structurally related to the death inducing decoy receptors DR4 and DR5. DcR1 and DcR2 are postulated to serve as oncogenes due to their anti-apoptotic effects. In case of cervical cancer, there are number of cases that have shown the downregulation of decoy receptor expression by methylating DcR1 or DcR2 to obtain the advantage of growth [90, 91].

Apart from TNFs, the expression of hTERT in cervical cancer has been analyzed and 80–100% showed hTERT mRNA expression [92]. hTERT promoter has a high GC content with CpG island that could be affected by the methylation in regulating its expression. Hypermethylation leads to decrement in the gene expression. More research related to this study is awaited for the future.

Tumour suppressor genes: There are several hypermethylated genes observed in invasive cancers with specific functions that get either silenced or diminished (**Table 2**). TSLC1 is the gene that code for Ig like intercellular adhesion molecule that is able to mediate the calcium-independent interactions of Ca2. It was first identified in lung cancer, and the reason of its silencing was derived from either the loss of

TSGs with rate of hypermethylation	Functions that get silenced or diminished
hTERT (57%)	apoptosis
P16 (8–42%)	Cell cycle
E-cadherin (28–81%)	WNT pathway
MGMT (5–81%)	DNA repair
BRAC1 (6.1%)	FA-BRAC pathway
TSLC1 (58–65%)	Tumour Suppressor
RASSF1A(0–45%)	Negative Ras effect
RAR beta (33–66%)	Cell differentiation
TIMP2/TIMP3 (47%)	Tissue inhibitor

Table 2.
Hypermethylated genes silenced or diminished by various pathways

heterozygosity or promoter hypermethylation. The effect of this gene in suppressing cervical cancer was demonstrated by the study related to transfection of TSLC1 cDNA to SiHa cells. It showed reduction in anchorage-independent growth and able to generate less tumours in nude mice. The cervical lesions are accompanied by the expression loss of this tumour suppressor gene as in a case study, it was observed to show 58–65% increment in methylation rate in invasive tumours.

For the regulation of epithelial cell differentiation, retinoic acid is essential which is mediated by the RA-binding nuclear receptors. The target genes transcriptions by ligand-activated receptors are induced by the binding of RA responsive elements in promoter regions. RAR beta gene is one of those target genes that encode for tumour suppression. In many tumour cell lines and human tumours in primary stages, the complete or partial inhibition of gene expression has been observed [93]. The hypermethylation of promoter in colon and breast cancer leading to inhibition of RAR beta 2 inhibition has been observed. The retinoic acid inhibits the human keratinocyte transcription by HPV 16 that leads to regression of cancer [94]. The methylation rate of RAR beta 2 gene has been observed to show the increment from 33 to 63% in invasive cancers [95].

Histone acetylation: The regulation of gene transcription is majorly performed by the balance between histone deacetylases and histone acetyl transferase activity. Thus, the proper balance should be maintained in order to check the cell proliferation. HPV has E6 and E7 oncoproteins that are responsible to cause disturbance in the cell growth and proliferation. The E7 protein binds to HDACs and forms Mi2beta, an intermediary protein from nucleosome remodelling and histone deacetylation (NURD) complex that could modify the structure of chromatin. This modification is done by the nucleosome repositioning and histone deacetylation. Any mutation to E7 abolishes its binding to HDAC1 that results in loss of E7 to transform rodent fibroblast. In cervical cancer, phosphorylated and acetylated forms of H3 in the smears have shown the association of its modification with the progression of lesions from CNI to CNIII [96].

15. Current treatment and diagnosis

Cancer is caused by damage or mutations in the genetic material of the cells as a result of environmental or hereditary factors. Anti-cancer drugs (chemotherapy, hormone therapy and biological therapies) are the treatment of choice for metastatic tumours, while surgery and radiation are the primary treatments for local and non-metastatic cancers. Chemotherapy works by preventing malignant cells from dividing quickly, but it also affects normal cells with fast proliferation rates, such as hair follicles, bone marrow and gastrointestinal tract cells, resulting in chemotherapy's typical side effects.

There is a growing need for new effective targeted treatments based on the molecular biology of tumour cells due to the indiscriminate destruction of normal cells, the toxic side effects of conventional chemotherapy and the emergence of multidrug resistance.

During the past few years, FDA-approved targeted cancer drugs have become increasingly popular, causing cancer cells to die via apoptosis or by stimulating the immune system. These novel targeted therapies are gaining momentum as indicated by the growing number of cancer drugs approved by the FDA.

There are a variety of cancer treatments available. Treatment options will vary based on the type of cancer that an individual has and how far it has progressed.

Some cancer patients will just require one treatment. Most people, however, receive a combination of treatments, such as surgery along with chemotherapy and radiation. When it comes to cancer treatment, there is a lot to learn and consider.

16. Cancer treatment biomarker testing

Biomarker testing is a method of looking for cancer-related genes, proteins and other chemicals (also known as biomarkers or tumour markers). Biomarker testing can assist an individual or doctor in determining the best cancer treatment option.

16.1 Chemotherapy

Chemotherapy is a cancer treatment that involves the administration of chemicals to kill cancer cells. Chemotherapy is a cancer treatment that is used in conjunction with other cancer treatments. It has negative effects and is used to fight cancer.

16.2 Hormone therapy

Hormone therapy is a type of treatment that slows or stops the progression of tumours that use hormones to grow, such as breast and prostate cancer.

16.3 Hyperthermia

Hyperthermia is a method of treatment in which bodily tissue is heated to temperatures as high as 113 degrees Fahrenheit in order to destroy and kill cancer cells while causing little or no injury to healthy tissue. Hyperthermia is used to treat different types of malignancies and precancers.

16.4 Immunotherapy

Immunotherapy is a cancer treatment that boosts your immune system's ability to fight cancer. The different types of immunotherapy are used to treat cancer,

16.5 Photodynamic therapy (PDT)

To eliminate cancer and other aberrant cells, photodynamic treatment uses a medication that is activated by light. Individual gets know how it works, the types of tumours and precancers it treats and the benefits and cons of this treatment.

16.6 Radiation therapy

Radiation therapy is a cancer treatment that involves administering high doses of radiation to cancer cells in order to kill them and shrink tumours. Individual gets to know about the many forms of radiation, its side effects, which side effects one might have and more.

16.7 Stem cell transplant

Stem cell transplants are treatments that replace stem cells in persons whose blood cells have been damaged by severe doses of chemotherapy or radiation therapy. Although there are several types of transplants and their possible adverse effects, stem cell transplants are currently employed in cancer treatment.

16.8 Surgery

Surgery is a procedure in which a surgeon removes cancer from the body to treat cancer. There are various ways in which surgery is used to treat cancer.

16.9 Targeted therapy

Targeted therapy is a cancer treatment that focuses on the modifications that help cancer cells grow, divide and spread. Individual can learn how therapy works against cancer and how to avoid the most common side effects.

17. miRNA as a diagnostic biomarker

The study of miRNA expression levels in tumours could aid in the identification of tumour types and subtypes, as well as the prediction of their characteristics. Several studies have proven that miRNAs can be used as prognostic and/or diagnostic tools in various malignancies. The study of miRNA expression levels in tumours could aid in the identification of tumour types and subtypes, as well as the prediction of their characteristics.

Lu and colleagues investigated the relationship between miRNA expression profiles and developmental origin in 334 samples from multiple human cancers. They found that miRNA expression profiles correlate with development of cancer tissues [97].

Cancers such as breast, colorectal, prostate and colorectal occur frequently as a consequence of incorrect expression of genes such as ANRIL, HOTAIR, KCNQ1OT1 and XIST 16.

18. The epigenetic changes in cancer diagnosis and treatment

DNA methylation and histone modifications are significant epigenetic processes of gene regulation that play important roles in tumour initiation and development, both individually and cooperatively. In prostate cancer, abnormal epigenetic processes such as DNA hypo- and hypermethylation, as well as altered histone acetylation, have been found, affecting a large number of genes. Although the number of abnormally epigenetically regulated genes continues to grow, only a few genes have shown promise as potential tumour biomarkers for prostate cancer early detection and risk assessment. To detect prostate cancer-specific epigenetic fingerprints, large-scale screening of aberrant epigenetic processes such as DNA hypermethylation is required [98]. In human malignancies, DNA methylation is the epigenetic mark that has been examined the most. In 1983, cancer-related DNA methylation was discovered. DNA methylation inhibitors were clinically used to treat a range of cancers within 30 years of their discovery, emphasizing the importance of the epigenetic basis of cancer. Histone alterations, nucleosome remodelling and microRNA (miRNA)-mediated gene regulation are all important in tumour development. In all stages of lung cancer, including start, development and metastasis, distinct chromatin changes occur. As a result, stage-specific epigenetic modifications can be used as powerful and reliable methods for lung cancer early detection and patient prognosis monitoring. Furthermore, chromatin modifiers are interesting targets for the development of more effective therapeutic techniques against epigenetic alterations since they are dynamic and reversible [99].

19. Phytochemicals involved in cancer treatment

Vinca alkaloids, taxane diterpenoids, camptothecin derivatives and epipodophyllotoxin are the four principal types of clinically employed plant-derived anticancer agents. Other plant-derived anticancer drugs, such as combretastatins, homoharringtonine (omacetaxine mepesuccinate, cephalotaxine alkaloid) and ingenol mebutate, are employed in addition to these phytochemical groups. Poor water solubility and considerable hazardous side effects are still key concerns, so researchers are currently focusing their efforts on reducing their impact. Several analogues and prodrugs have been created in this context, as well as approaches to improve aqueous solubility and tumour selectivity. Below is a brief summary of a few phytochemicals that are employed in cancer treatment.

19.1 Vinca alkaloids

Vinca alkaloids are a class of medications derived from *Catharanthus roseus*, a pink periwinkle plant. The Vinca alkaloids cause cytotoxicity by binding to tubulin at a different position than the taxanes, preventing microtubule polymerization and assembly, resulting in metaphase arrest and cell death. The vinca alkaloids influence both malignant and non-malignant cells in the non-mitotic cell cycle because microtubules are involved in various other cellular processes such as cell shape preservation, motility and transfer between organelles. The two naturally separated alkaloids vinblastine and vincristine have been utilized in clinical oncology for nearly 50 years. These two alkaloids have a number of semisynthetic equivalents that have been produced. Vinorelbine and vindesine are two semisynthetic analogues that have been approved for use in clinical trials. These drugs are commonly used in combination chemotherapy to treat a range of cancers [100].

19.2 Taxanes

Taxanes are anticancer compounds that were first discovered in the bark of the Yew tree. Taxanes inhibit cancer growth by stabilizing microtubules, causing cell cycle arrest and abnormal mitosis. Paclitaxel, a natural substance derived from the bark and leaves of Taxus brevifolia and docetaxel, a semi-synthetic derivative, are largely used in the treatment of breast, ovarian, pancreatic, prostate and lung cancers. A number of semisynthetic compounds with better cytotoxicity in resistant tumours, reduced toxicity and improved solubility have been produced. Cabazitaxel, a second-generation docetaxel derivative, for example, has cytotoxic effectiveness against a variety of docetaxel-resistant cancers while posing a lower overall toxicity risk

[101, 102]. Cabazitaxel also has the ability to permeate the blood-brain barrier in vivo, which is something that other taxanes can't do. Larotaxel, milataxel, ortataxel and tesetaxel are some of the paclitaxel analogues now being studied in clinical trials.

19.3 Camptothecins

Camptothecin is a quinolone alkaloid discovered from *Camptotheca acuminata*, a Chinese tree. Camptothecin forms a compound with type I DNA topoisomerase, which prevents DNA cleavage and religation, resulting in a DNA double-strand break and cytotoxicity [103]. Currently, the two FDA-approved semi-synthetic camptothecin derivatives that are therapeutically active and less toxic than the parent molecule are irinotecan and topotecan. Irinotecan is a drug that is used to treat advanced malignancies of the gut and rectum. Topotecan, on the other hand, has been approved for the treatment of ovarian cancer, small-cell lung cancer and cervical cancer.

19.4 Podophyllotoxins

Podophyllotoxin is a naturally occurring toxin found in the plants *Podophyllum peltatum and Podophyllum emodi* (Berberidaceae). Podophyllotoxin binds to tubulin in a reversible manner, whereas its main derivatives etoposide and teniposide inhibit topoisomerase II, causing DNA cleavage by topoisomerase II. Furthermore, podophyllotoxin has anti-multidrug resistance (MDR) efficacy against a variety of drug-resistant tumour cells. CIP-36, a podophyllotoxin derivative, has been found to overcome the MDR of the adriamycin-resistant K562/ADR human leukaemic cell line by modulating topoisomerase-IIa activity [104]. CIP-36, on the other hand, failed in clinical testing due to ineffectiveness and unacceptable toxicity.

19.5 Reversal of hypermethylation

Lee et al. also discovered that EGCG and similar substances inhibit DNMT and reverse hypermethylation [105, 106]. They discovered that EGCG inhibited DNMT activity directly and partially altered the methylation state of RAR-ß. Other catechol polyphenols inhibited DNMT indirectly by methylating S-adenosyl-L-methionine (SAM) and converting it to S-adenosyl-L-homocysteine (SAH), a potent DNMT inhibitor. In breast cancer cell lines, caffeic acid and chlorogenic acid partially prevented methylation of the RAR-ß gene promoter region [106]. The effect of EGCG, however, may be gene or cell line specific, and it was not as strong as 5-aza-2′-deoxycytidine (DAC) [107].

Some of the methylation-silenced genes were discovered to be demethylated and reactivated by isoflavones, with genistein being the most effective isoflavone from soy [108]. Genistein (20–50 mmol/L) suppressed DNMT activity in a dose-dependent manner, with competitive and noncompetitive inhibition of the substrate. Biochanin A and daidzein, two other isoflavones, were less effective in inhibiting DNMT activity, reactivating RAR- and stopping cancer cell growth. Although genistein was a weaker DNMT inhibitor than EGCG, it was equally as effective or even more effective than EGCG in demethylating hypermethylated genes and reactivating their expression.

When KYSE 510 cells were treated with 2 M genistein and 5 M EGCG, or 5 M genistein and 10 M EGCG, the expression of p16 was apparently increased compared with genistein or EGCG alone. The synergistic activity of these two drugs raised the levels of acetylated histone H3 and H4 in KYSE 510 cells when they were treated with genistein (5 M) for 5 days and subsequently with the HDAC inhibitor trichostatin (0.5 M) for 3 hours. Genistein and trichostatin increase the binding of acetylated H3 and H4 to the promoter region of RAR- and MGMT in a synergistic manner, according to a chromatin immunoprecipitation (ChIP) test. Other dietary components that inhibit DNMT include quercetin, luteolin, and hydroxycinnamic acid.

20. Conclusion

In the reports of 2018, 18.1 million new cancer cases were detected with 53% mortality rate. This disease is more prevalent in males as compared in females with ratio of 1.17. There are about more than 100 types of cancers that have been reported. Cancer is the disease that is caused by the genetic and the epigenetic factors that cause alterations in the gene functions. These genes are known as tumour suppressor genes which perform crucial function in inhibiting the invasion of tumour and its progression in the cell. The epigenetic factors such as hypomethylation in oncogenes, hypermethylation of tumour suppressor genes and the direct mutagenesis. These epigenetic factors are responsible for the tumorigenesis, and they are reversible in nature which makes them different from the genetic mutations. The new need of targeted molecular therapy is required on tumour cells as they are different from the normal cells, but the old treatments of cancer by radiotherapy and chemotherapy have the toxic side effect with less survival rate. The reversal could be done by the phytochemicals. There are various phytochemicals known that have shown the apoptosis in cancer cells such as alkaloid, taxane, camptothecins and podophyllotxins. These phytochemicals such as EGCG have been observed to inhibit the activity of DNMT1 directly and the partial activity of the rar-beta gene. In some cases, isoflavones have been observed to demethylate and reactivate the suppressor genes. The phytochemicals could be used as a drug to treat and prevent cancer by reversing the promoter hypermethylated genes that lead to loss of vital function performing genes such as transcriptional factors. These epigenetic factors could be used in future research to identify, diagnose, prevent and treat cancer as they could serve as one of the primary hallmarks of cancer and the reversal could lead to early prevention of cancer.

21. Future prospects

The epigenetic factors involved in the cancer could be either aberrant methylation (hypomethylation or hypermethylation) or direct mutagenesis of the vital genes. The genes that play a vital role in suppression of tumorigenesis, when altered by the epigenetic factors, lose their function such as gatekeeper genes or transcription factors. These epigenetic factors could be used as primary hallmark for the early detection of cancer. The DNA aberrant methylation could be reversed by the phytochemicals and be used in early-stage treatment of cancer. Thus, these epigenetic factors that lead to cancer and tumorigenesis can play a vital role in early diagnosis, prevention and treatment of this disease.

Author details

Mehak Sharan[1], Runjhun Mathur[1,2], Niraj Kumar Jha[1], Khushboo Rana[1], Saurabh Kumar Jha[1] and Abhimanyu Kumar Jha[1*]

1 Department of Biotechnology, Sharda University, Greater Noida, Uttar Pradesh, India

2 Dr. A.P.J Abdul Kalam Technical University, Lucknow, Uttar Pradesh, India

*Address all correspondence to: abhimanyujha630@gmail.com

References

[1] Hajdu SI. A note from history: Landmarks in history of cancer, part 1. Cancer. 2011;**117**(5):1097-1102

[2] Paul of Aegina, 7th Century AD, quoted in Moss, Ralph W. "Galen on Cancer." Cancer Decisions. Archived from the original on 16 July 2011. Referenced from Michael Shimkin, Contrary to Nature, Washington, DC: Superintendent of Document, DHEW Publication No. (NIH). 2004. 79–720, p. 35

[3] Hajdu SI. A note from history: Landmarks in history of cancer, part 2. Cancer. 2011;**117**(12):2811-2820

[4] Yalom M. A History of the Breast. 1st ed. New York: Ballantine Books; 1998

[5] "Cancer". World Health Organization. 12 September 2018. Retrieved 19 December 2018

[6] Cancer – Signs and symptoms. NHS Choices. Archived from the original on 8 June 2014. Retrieved 10 June 2014

[7] "Defining Cancer". National Cancer Institute. 17 September 2007. Retrieved 28 March 2018

[8] Anand P, Kunnumakkara AB, Sundaram C, Harikumar KB, Tharakan ST, Lai OS, et al. Cancer is a preventable disease that requires major lifestyle changes. Pharmaceutical Research. 2008; **25**(9):2097-2116

[9] World Cancer Report 2014. World Health Organization. 2014. pp. Chapter 1.1. ISBN: 978-92-832-0429-9. Archived from the original on 12 July 2017

[10] "Heredity and Cancer". American Cancer Society. Archived from the original on 2 August 2013. Retrieved 22 July 2013

[11] Kushi LH, Doyle C, McCullough M, Rock CL, Demark-Wahnefried W, Bandera EV, et al. American Cancer Society Guidelines on nutrition and physical activity for cancer prevention: Reducing the risk of cancer with healthy food choices and physical activity. CA: A Cancer Journal for Clinicians Cancer. 2012;**62**(1):30-67

[12] Parkin DM, Boyd L, Walker LC (December 2011). "16. The fraction of cancer attributable to lifestyle and environmental factors in the UK in 2010". British Journal of Cancer 105 Suppl 2: S77–S81

[13] World Cancer Report 2014. World Health Organization. 2014. pp. Chapter 4.7. ISBN: 978-92-832-0429-9. Archived from the original on 12 July 2017

[14] "SEER Stat Fact Sheets: All Cancer Sites." National Cancer Institute. Archived from the original on 26 September 2010. Retrieved 18 June 2014

[15] Islami F, Goding Sauer A, Miller KD, Siegel RL, Fedewa SA, Jacobs EJ, et al. Proportion and number of cancer cases and deaths attributable to potentially modifiable risk factors in the United States. CA: A Cancer Journal for Clinicians. 2018;**68**(1):31-54

[16] Cohen S, Murphy ML, Prather AA. Ten surprising facts about stressful life events and disease risk. Annual Review of Psychology. 2019;**70**:577-597

[17] Heikkilä K, Nyberg ST, Theorell T, Fransson EI, Alfredsson L, Bjorner JB, et al. "Work stress and risk of cancer: Meta-analysis of 5700 incident cancer events in 116,000 European men and women". 2013

[18] "Latest global cancer data: Cancer burden rises to 18.1 million new cases

and 9.6 million cancer deaths in 2018" (PDF)

[19] Ward E, DeSantis C, Robbins A, Kohler B, Jemal A. Childhood and adolescent cancer statistics, 2014. CA: A Cancer Journal for Clinicians. 2014;**64** (2):83-103

[20] Fathallah-Shaykh HM, Zhao LJ, Mickey B, Kafrouni AI. Molecular advances to treat cancer of the brain. Expert Opinion on Investigational Drugs. 2000;**9**(6):1207-1215

[21] Smalley M, Ashworth A. Stem cells and breast cancer: A field in transit. Nature Reviews. Cancer. 2003;**3**(11): 832-844

[22] Vargo-Gogola T, Rosen JM. Modelling breast cancer: One size does not fitall. Nature Reviews. Cancer. 2007; **7**(9):659-672

[23] Burghardt E. Early histological diagnosis of cervical cancer. Major Problems in Obstetrics and Gynecology. 1973;**6**:1-401

[24] Hofmeister S. Cervical cancer screening: How our approach may change. The Journal of Family Practice. 2016;**65**(8):551-553

[25] Marley AR, Nan H. Epidemiology of colorectal cancer. International Journal of Molecular Epidemiology and Genetics. 2016;**7**(3):10514

[26] Enzinger PC, Mayer RJ. Esophageal cancer. The New England Journal of Medicine. 2003;**349**(23):2241-2252

[27] Napier KJ, Scheerer M, Misra S. Esophageal cancer: A review of epidemiology, pathogenesis, staging workup and treatment modalities. World Journal of Gastrointestinal Oncology. 2014;**6**(5):112-120

[28] Van der Schroeff MP, Baatenburg de Jong RJ. Staging and prognosis in head and neck cancer. Oral Oncology. 2009; **45**(4–5):356-360

[29] Popescu B, Ene P, Bertesteanu SV, et al. Methods of investigating metastatic lymph nodes in head and neck cancer. Maedica. 2013;**8**(4):384-387

[30] Glazer CA, Chang SS, Ha PK, et al. Applying the molecular biology and epigenetics of head and neck cancer in everyday clinical practice. Oral Oncology. 2009;**45**(4–5):440-446

[31] Báez A. Genetic and environmental factors in head and neck cancer genesis. Journal of Environmental Science and Health. Part C, Environmental Carcinogenesis & Ecotoxicology Reviews. 2008;**26**(2):174-200

[32] Hui JY. Epidemiology and etiology of sarcomas. Surgical Clinical of North America. 2016;**96**(5):901-914; Cairns P. Renal cell carcinoma. Cancer Biomarkers 2010;9(1–6):461–73

[33] Sudarshan S, Linehan WM. Genetic basis of cancer of the kidney. Seminars in Oncology. 2006;**33**(5):544-551

[34] Sidana A, Srinivasan R. Therapeutic strategies for hereditary kidney cancer. Current Oncology Reports. 2016; **18**(8):50

[35] Zhi XS, Xiong J, Zi XY, Hu YP. The potential role of liver stem cells in initiation of primary liver cancer. Hepatology International. 2016;**10**(6): 893-901

[36] Tsukuma H, Tanaka H, Ajiki W, Oshima A. Liver cancer and its prevention. Asian Pacific Journal of Cancer Prevention. 2005;**6**(3): 244-250

[37] Sánchez-Aguilera A, Méndez-Ferrer S. The hematopoietic stem-cell niche in health and leukemia. Cellular and Molecular Life Sciences. 2016;**74**(4): 579-590

[38] Knudson AG. Two genetic hits (more or less) to cancer. Nature Reviews. Cancer. 2001;**1**:157-162

[39] Baylin SB, Jones PA. A decade of exploring the cancer epigenome—Biological and translational implications. Nature Reviews. Cancer. 2011;**11**:726-734

[40] You JS, Jones PA. Cancer genetics and epigenetics: Two sides of the same coin? Cancer Cell. 2012;**22**:9-20

[41] Reddy KL, Feinberg AP. Higher order chromatin organization in cancer. Seminars in Cancer Biology. 2013;**23**: 109-115

[42] Bernstein BE, Stamatoyannopoulos JA, Costello JF, Ren B, Milosavljevic A, Meissner A, et al. The NIH Roadmap epigenomics mapping consortium. Nature Biotechnology. 2010;**28**: 1045-1048

[43] Zheng L, Dai H, Zhou M, Li X, Liu C, Guo Z, et al. Polyploid cells rewire DNA damage response networks to overcome replication stress-induced barriers for tumour progression. Nature Communications. 2012;**3**:815

[44] Jones PA, Laird PW. Cancer epigenetics comes of age. Nature Genetics. 1999;**21**:163-167

[45] Ehrlich M, Lacey M. DNA hypomethylation and hemimethylation in cancer. Advances in Experimental Medicine and Biology. 2013;**754**:31-56

[46] Chen RZ, Pettersson U, Beard C, Jackson-Grusby L, Jaenisch R. DNA hypomethylation leads to elevated mutation rates. Nature. 1998;**395**:89-93

[47] Greenblatt MS, Bennett WP, Hollstein M, Harris CC. Mutations in the p53 tumor suppressor gene: Clues to cancer etiology and molecular pathogenesis. Cancer Research. 1994;**54**: 4855-4878

[48] Jones PA, Baylin SB. The epigenomics of cancer. Cell. 2007;**128**: 683-692

[49] Kulis M, Heath S, Bibikova M, Queiros AC, Navarro A, Clot G, et al. Epigenomic analysis detects widespread gene-body DNA hypomethylation in chronic lymphocytic leukemia. Nature Genetics. 2012;**44**:1236-1242

[50] Egger G, Liang G, Aparicio A, Jones PA. Epigenetics in human disease and prospects for epigenetic therapy. Nature. 2004;**429**:457-463

[51] Baylin SB, Herman JG. DNA hypermethylation in tumorigenesis: Epigenetics joins genetics. Trends in Genetics. 2000;**16**:168-174

[52] Jones PA, Laird PW. Cancer epigenetics comes of age. Nature Genetics. 1999;**21**:163-167

[53] Costello JF, Fruhwald MC, Smiraglia DJ, et al. Aberrant CpG-island methylation has non-random and tumor-type-specific patterns. Nature Genetics. 2000;**24**:132-138

[54] Toyota M, Ho C, Ahuja N, et al. Identification of differentially methylated sequences in colorectal cancer by methylated CpG island amplification. Cancer Research. 1999;**59**: 2307-2312

[55] Toyota M, Ahuja N, Ohe-Toyota M, Herman JG, Baylin SB, Issa JP. CpG

island methylator phenotype in colorectal cancer. Proceedings of the National Academy of Science USA. 1999; **96**:8681-8686

[56] Baylin SB, Belinsky SA, Herman JG. Aberrant methylation of gene promoters in cancer—concepts, misconcepts and promise. Journal of the National Cancer Institute. 2000;**92**:1460-1461

[57] Makos M, Nelkin BD, Lerman MI, Latif F, Zbar B, Baylin SB. Distinct hypermethylation patterns occur at altered chromosome loci in human lung and colon cancer. Proceedings of the National Academy of Science USA. 1992; **89**:1929-1933

[58] Wales MM, Biel MA, el Deiry W, et al. p53 activates expression of HIC-1, a new candidate tumour suppressor gene on 17p13.3. Nature Medicine. 1995;**1**: 570-577

[59] Makos M, Nelkin BD, Reiter RE, et al. Regional DNA hypermethylation at D17S5 precedes 17p structural changes in the progression of renal tumors. Cancer Research. 1993;**53**:2719-2722

[60] Guerardel C, Deltour S, Pinte S, et al. Identification in the human candidate tumor suppressor gene HIC-1 of a new major alternative TATA-less promoter positively regulated by p53. The Journal of Biological Chemistry. 2001;**275**:307-308

[61] Carter MG, Johns MA, Zeng X, et al. Mice deficient in the candidate tumor suppressor gene Hic1 exhibit developmental defects of structures affected in the Miller–Dieker syndrome. Human Molecular Genetics. 2000;**9**: 413-419

[62] Foster SA, Wong DJ, Barrett MT, Galloway DA. Inactivation of p16 in human mammary epithelial cells by CpG island methylation. Molecular and Cellular Biology. 1998;**18**:1793-1801

[63] Loughran O, Malliri A, Owens D, et al. Association of CDKN2A/p16INK4A with human head and neck keratinocyte replicative senescence: Relationship of dysfunction to immortality and neoplasia. Oncogene. 1996;**13**:561-568

[64] Wong DJ, Barrett MT, Stoger R, Emond MJ, Reid BJ. p16INK4a promoter is hypermethylated at a high frequency in esophageal adenocarcinomas. Cancer Research. 1997;**57**:2619-2622

[65] Belinsky SA, Nikula KJ, Palmisano WA, et al. Aberrant methylation of p16 (INK4a) is an early event in lung cancer and a potential biomarker for early diagnosis. Proceedings of the National Academy of Science USA. 1998;**95**: 11891-11896

[66] Kinzler KW, Vogelstein B. Cancer-susceptibility genes. Gatekeepers and caretakers. Nature. 1997;**386**:761-763

[67] Graff JR, Gabrielson E, Fujii H, Baylin SB, Herman JG. Methylation patterns of the E-cadherin 5′ CpG island are unstable and reflect the dynamic, heterogeneous loss of E-cadherin expression during metastatic progression. The Journal of Biological Chemistry. 2000;**275**:2727-2732

[68] Pietenpol JA, Bohlander SK, Sato Y, et al. Assignment of the human p27Kip1 gene to 12p13 and its analysis in leukemias. Cancer Research. 1995;**55**: 1206-1210

[69] Hsieh CL. Dependence of transcriptional repression on CpG methylation density. Molecular and Cellular Biology. 1994;**14**:5487-5494

[70] Vertino PM, Yen RW, Gao J, Baylin SB. De novo methylation of CpG island

sequences in human fibroblasts overexpressing DNA (cytosine-5-)-methyltransferase. Molecular and Cellular Biology. 1996;**16**: 4555-4565

[71] Myohanen SK, Baylin SB, Herman JG. Hypermethylation can selectively silence individual p16ink4A alleles in neoplasia. Cancer Research. 1998;**58**: 591-593

[72] Mareel M, Bracke M, Van Roy F. CaNcer metastasis: Negative regulation by an invasion-suppressor complex. Cancer Detection and Prevention. 1995; **19**:451-464

[73] Moll R, Mitze M, Frixen UH, Birchmeier W. Differential loss of E-cadherin expression in infiltrating ductal and lobular breast carcinomas. The American Journal of Pathology. 1993; **143**:1731-1742

[74] Siitonen SM, Kononen JT, Helin HJ, Rantala IS, Holli KA, Isola JJ. Reduced E-cadherin expression is associated with invasiveness and unfavorable prognosis in breast cancer. American Journal of Clinical Pathology. 1996;**105**:394-402

[75] Cameron EE, Bachman KE, Myohanen S, Herman JG, Baylin SB. Synergy of demethylation and histone deacetylase inhibition in the re-expression of genes silenced in cancer. Nature Genetics. 1999;**21**:103-107

[76] Cairns J. Mutation selection and the natural history of cancer. Nature. 1975; **255**:197-200

[77] Fearon ER, Vogelstein, 8. A genetic model for colorectal tumorigenesis. Cell. 1990;**61**:759-767

[78] Harris H. The analysis of malignancy by cell fusion: The position in 1988. Cancer Research. 1988;**48**:3302-3306

[79] Stanbridge EJ, Ceredig R. Growth-regulatory control of human cell hybrids in nude mice. Cancer Research. 1981;**47**: 573-580

[80] "Tumor Suppressor (TS) Genes and the Two-Hit Hypothesis | Learn Science at Scitable". www.nature.com. Retrieved 2019-10-06

[81] Harris CC. Structure and function of p53 tumor suppressor gene: Clues for rational cancer therapeutic strategies. Journal of the National Cancer Institute. 1996;**88**(20):1442-1455. DOI: 10.1093/jnci/88.20.1442. PMID 8841019

[82] "BCL2 (B-Cell Leukemia/ Lymphoma 2)." atlasgeneticsoncology. org. Retrieved 2019-11-21

[83] Antequera F, Bird A. CpG islands. EXS. 1993;**64**:169-185

[84] Verma M. Viral genes and methylation. Annals of the New York Academy of Sciences. 2003;**983**:170-180

[85] Tao Q, Huang H, Geiman TM, Lim CY, Fu L, Qiu GH, et al. Defective de novo methylation of viral and cellular DNA sequences in ICF syndrome cells. Human Molecular Genetics. 2002;**11**: 2091-2102. DOI: 10.1093/hmg/ 11.18.2091

[86] Tao Q, Robertson KD. Stealth technology: How Epstein-Barr virus utilizes DNA methylation to cloak itself from immune detection. Clinical Immunology. 2003;**109**:53-63. DOI: 10.1016/S1521-6616(03)00198-0

[87] Rosl F, Arab A, Klevenz B, zur Hausen H. The effect of DNA methylation on gene regulation of human papillomaviruses. The Journal of General Virology. 1993;**74**:791-801

[88] Kalantari M, Calleja-Macías IE, Tewari D, Hagmar B, Lie K, Barrera-Saldaña HA, et al. Conserved methylation patterns of human papillomavirus type 16 DNA in asymptomatic infection and cervical neoplasia. Journal of Virology. 2004;**78**: 12762-12772

[89] Thain A, Jenkins O, Clarke AR, Gaston K. CpG methylation directly inhibits binding of the human papillomavirus type 16 E2 protein to specific DNA sequences. Journal of Virology. 1996;**70**:7233-7235

[90] Van Noesel MM, van Bezouw S, Salomons GS, Voute PA, Pieters R, Baylin SB, et al. Tumor-specific down-regulation of the tumor necrosis factor-related apoptosis-inducing ligand decoy receptors DcR1 and DcR2 is associated with dense promoter hypermethylation. Cancer Research. 2002;**62**:2157-2161

[91] Ashkenazi A, Dixit VM. Apoptosis control by death and decoy receptors. Current Opinion in Cell Biology. 1999;**11**: 255-260

[92] Ozoren N, El-Deiry WS. Cell surface death receptor signaling in normal and cancer cells. Seminars in Cancer Biology. 2003;**13**:135-147

[93] Nakano N, Watney E, McDougall JK. Telomerase activity and expression of telomerase RNA component and telomerase catalytic subunit gene in cervical cancer. The American Journal of Pathology. 1998;**153**:857-864

[94] Chambon P. The retinoid signaling pathway: Molecular and genetic analyses. Seminars in Cell Biology. 1994; **5**:115-125

[95] Meyskens FL, Surwit E, Moon TE, Childers JM, Davis JR, Dorr RT, et al. Enhancement of regression of cervical intraepithelial neoplasia II (moderate dysplasia) with topically applied all-trans retinoic acid: A randomized trial. Journal of the National Cancer Institute. 1994;**86**:539-543

[96] Vanova T, Petrenko A, Gritsko T, Vinokourova S, Eshilev E, Kobzeva V, et al. Methylation and silencing of the retinoic acid receptor-beta 2 gene in cervical cancer. BMC Cancer. 2002;**2**:4

[97] Visone R, Croce CM. MiRNAs and cancer. The American Journal of Pathology. 2009;**174**:1131-1138

[98] Li L-C, Carroll PR, Dahiya R. Epigenetic changes in prostate cancer: Implication for diagnosis and treatment. National Cancer Institute. 2005;**97**(2): 103-115

[99] Mehta A, Dobersch S, Romero-Olmedo AJ, Barreto G. Epigenetics in lung cancer diagnosis and therapy. Cancer Metastasis Review. 2015;**34**(2): 229-241

[100] Martino E, Casamassima G, Castiglione S, Cellupica E, Pantalone S, Papagni F, et al. Vinca alkaloids and analogues as anti-cancer agents: Looking back, peering ahead. Bioorganic & Medicinal Chemistry Letters. 2018;**28** (17):2816-2826. DOI: 10.1016/j.bmcl.2018.06.044

[101] Kotsakis A, Matikas A, Koinis F, Kentepozidis N, Varthalitis II, Karavassilis V, et al. A multicentre phase II trial of cabazitaxel in patients with advanced non-small-cell lung cancer progressing after docetaxel-based chemotherapy. British Journal of Cancer. 2016;**115**(7):784-788. DOI: 10.1038/bjc.2016.281

[102] Oudard S, Fizazi K, Sengelov L, Daugaard G, Saad F, Hansen S, et al. Cabazitaxel versus docetaxel as first-line

therapy for patients with metastatic castration-resistant prostate cancer: A randomized phase III trial-firstana. Journal of Clinical Oncology. 2017;**35**(28):3189-3197. DOI: 10.1200/JCO.2016.72.1068

[103] Hertzberg RP, Caranfa MJ, Hecht SM. On the mechanism of topoisomerase, I inhibition by camptothecin: Evidence for binding to an enzyme-DNA complex. Biochemistry. 1989;**28**(11):4629-4638. DOI: 10.1021/bi00437a018

[104] Cao B, Chen H, Gao Y, Niu C, Zhang Y, Li L. CIP-36, a novel topoisomerase II-targeting agent, induces the apoptosis of multidrug-resistant cancer cells in vitro. International Journal of Molecular Medicine. 2015;**35**(3):771-776. DOI: 10.3892/ijmm.2015.2068

[105] Lee WJ, Shim JY, Zhu BT. Mechanisms for the inhibition of DNA methyltransferases by tea catechins and bioflavonoids. Molecular Pharmacology. 2005;**68**:1018-1030

[106] Lee WJ, Zhu BT. Inhibition of DNA methylation by caffeic acid and chlorogenic acid, two common catechol-containing coffee polyphenols. Carcinogenesis. 2006;**27**:269-277

[107] Chuang JC, Yoo CB, Kwan JM, et al. Comparison of biological effects of non-nucleoside DNA methylation inhibitors versus 5-aza-2′-deoxycytidine. Molecular Cancer Therapeutics. 2005;**4**:1515-1520

[108] Fang MZ, Chen D, Sun Y, Jin Z, Christman JK, Yang CS. Reversal of hypermethylation and reactivation of p16INK4a, RARbeta, and MGMT genes by genistein and other isoflavones from soy. Clinical Cancer Research. 2005;**11**:7033-7041

Chapter 4

Role of NGS in Oral Squamous Cell Carcinoma

Sivapatham Sundaresan and Lavanya Selvaraj

Abstract

A recent advance next generation sequencing (NGS) technology has enabled the identification of potential disease-based biomarkers in saliva or epithelial cells. There has been no effective oral squamous cell carcinoma (OSCC) biomarker or well-organised molecular detection method until now, which make early diagnosis difficult, if not impossible. This chapter summarises advances in cancer research using NGS and proposes biomarkers for screening and diagnosis of OSCC using the NGS technique. As part of our review, we covered four categories: OSCC and salivary biomarkers, Uses of NGS and definitions, present biomarkers in NGS, and Candidate salivary biomarkers for OSCC using NGS.

Keywords: next generation sequencing, oral squamous cell carcinoma, biomarkers, cancer

1. Introduction

Oral cancer belongs to a larger subgroup of tumours termed head and neck cancer, comprising lip, mobile tongue, buccal, labial, floor of the mouth, gingiva, hard palate and soft palate [1]. Buccal malignancies most commonly arise on the buccal posterior-lateral border and ventral surfaces [2]. Squamous cell carcinoma of the oral epithelium accounts for approximately 90% of all oral malignancies. The other 10% are malignant intraoral salivary gland tumours, melanomas, soft tissue and jaw bone sarcomas, non-lymphomas, Hodgkin's and the extremely rare malignant odontogenic tumours, as well as metastatic tumours of primary cancers situated elsewhere in the body [3].

Oral cancer is the most frequent in India, accounting for 50–70% of global cancer mortality and having the highest prevalence within Asian countries [4]. With an estimated one percent of the population possessing oral premalignant lesions, India is fittingly dubbed "the mouth cancer capital of the world." Every year, nearly one million persons in India are diagnosed with oral cancer, and half of them die in agony within a year of diagnosis due to late presentation [5]. A small percentage of newly diagnosed mouth cancer patients survive for an extended period of time.

Squamous cell carcinoma accounts for 90% of malignant tumours in the oral mucosa. The prevalence of cancer varies greatly around the global. The United Kingdom and the United States, the rate of all forms of tumours is 4%, however it is nearly 40% in South-East Asian countries [6]. Squamous cell carcinoma could manifest in a variety of clinical presentations. The aim is to recognise it primary because this is a crucial element prompting the clinical prognosis of the patient, and therefore suspicion and vigilance are seen as crucial aspects in cancer diagnosis [7]. Early lesions rarely cause symptoms, however they might manifest as a minor exophytic growth with little erythema or ulceration, a small ulcer, or erythroplakia, a white patch [8]. In clinical terms, characteristics such as induration, ulceration, and tissue fixation to structures could raise the possibility of an primary cancer. A late stage lesion typically manifests as a wide-based protrusion with a nodular, rough, haemorrhagic, warty, or necrotic surface 20, but it can similarly manifest as a destructive crater-like ulcer with rolling, elevated evented borders [6]. Histology of oral squamous cell carcinoma reveals a variety of forms (**Figure 1**). Despite this, all types exhibit tissue damage and invasion. Squamous cell carcinoma is graded according to its histology into well, moderately, and moderately differentiated groups [8]. Plasma cells and lymphocytic cells are frequently found infiltrating the stroma and aiding the assaulting epithelium. Several tumours occupy with a wide anterior, whilst others are composed of tiny islands or solitary aggressive cells. Cohesive cancer has a broad aggressive anterior, whereas non-cohesive carcinoma has tiny islands or single cells that infiltrate. It have been discovered that non-cohesive assault has a poor prognosis. Vascular, neuronal, and bone invasion all can occur [9]. The metastatic range of cancer in regional lymph nodes is classified into two types: intracapsular spread (when the spread is limited to the node's capsule) and extracapsular spread (when the

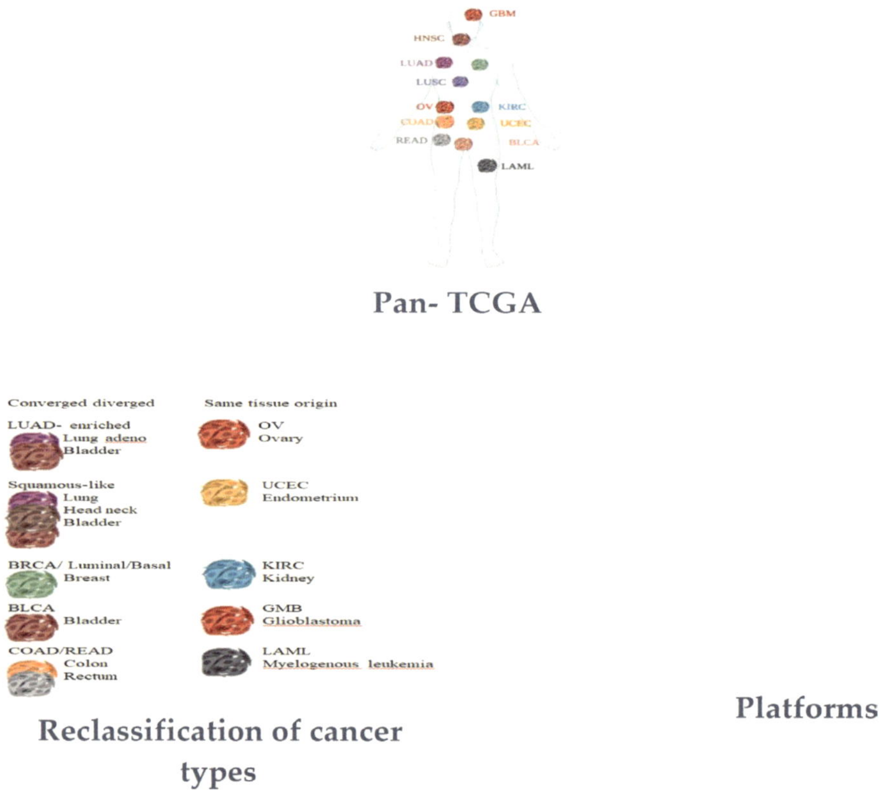

Figure 1.
A new cancer classification system could also have an impact on drug development and patient recruitment for clinical trials modified.

cancer spreads to neighbouring tissue near to the capsule). When the cancer develops extracapsular dissemination, the prognosis is poor [10].

2. Next-generation sequencing (NGS) and cancer

The concept of 'next-generation sequencing' (NGS) denotes to a range of knowledge that are viewed as the predecessors to the traditional Sanger DNA sequencing technique. Their advancement has enabled the generation of massive amounts of genomic data (almost one billion lines) at a low cost. This enables a wide range of applications, as well as whole-exome sequencing, whole-genome sequencing, including targeted gene sequencing [11]. Exome sequencing (the parts of DNA a certain encode proteins) is especially important from a scientific standpoint because it is believed that deviates in these areas account for around 85 percent of disease-causing mutations [12]. NGS has been used in numerous researchs to analyse the tumour exomes of samples from patients with head and neck SCC (HNSCC) [13]. Stransky et al. discovered a frequency of 130 coding mutations for each tumour and detected alterations in 39 recognised genes across the population studied [14], whereas Agrawal et al. discovered somatic mutations in genes previously linked to OSCC development. Both investigations also found substantial mutations in the signalling gene NOTCH1, that had not previously been linked to HNSC [15].

NGS can be used to analyse the RNA transcriptome in addition to DNA sequencing (RNA-Seq). The transcriptome is the complete set of transcribed RNA in a sample, and sequencing consents for both assessment of relative gene expression and identification of nucleotide polymorphisms [16]. Gene expression microarrays, which rely on the hybridisation and fluorescence of pre-designed probes, have been used in RNA expression studies till recently. Gene expression microarrays, that have well-developed molecular technology and a substantial body of research [17], have major advantages over RNA-Seq. For starters, RNA-Seq does not require a thorough understanding of the genes' targets, eliminating this need specialised probes. There is no limit to the number of genes that can be analysed simultaneously, unlike gene expression microarrays. Chromosomal translocations, fusion genes, differential splice variants, Single nucleotide polymorphisms, and viral transcripts are among the other transcriptome modifications that can be detected with RNA-Seq [18]. Tuch et al. discovered and proved with real-time quantitative reverse transcriptase polymerase chain reaction (RT-qPCR) that RNA-Seq was superior to gene expression microarray for identifying differential expression in transcripts with low expression levels in their investigation [19]. RNA-Seq has been used in a number of studies to investigate gene expression and transcriptome variation in various forms of HNSCC, including oral, oesophageal, and oropharyngeal. Quantification of differential gene expression, gene ontology analysis to identify over-represented, under-represented, and dysregulated biochemical mechanisms, classification of chromosomal translocations and subsequent fusion genes, attribution of differentially expressed novel mRNA splice variants, and investigation for HPV and other viral mRNA transcripts are all demonstrated applications of RNA-Seq in these studies. The Life TechnologiesTM (Carlsbad, USA) Ion ProtonTM/ Ion Personal Genome MachineTM (PGM) system is an NGS platform that uses proton release associated with Gene polymerisation to identify nucleotide sequence (ion semiconductor sequencing). Clonally amplified DNA fragments are challenged with free nucleotides in micro-machined wells equipped with pH sensors. The incorporation of nucleotides results in the release of a proton, resulting in a detectable pH shift.

This process is continued with each nucleotide cycle, resulting in the formation of a DNA sequence [20]. Ion semiconductor sequencing is quicker and less costly than other NGS technologies, however it has a shorter read length and a greater error rate. It has, however, been proved to be accurate in detecting nucleotide polymorphism.

Recent genomics studies are focusing on the molecular alterations that underpin the development of HNSCC and OSCC from both the epithelial and immunological compartments. These it has been shown that HNSCC and OSCC are extremely diverse, and despite the paucity of identifiable oncogenic mutations, targetable signalling pathways have been found. Furthermore, developing data from these research can be used to subclassify patients, for example, to those who may be more receptive to immunotherapies. Despite the fact that the majority of these have generated promising therapeutic effects, significant work remains to be done to expand the pharmacological arsenal available to OSCC patients. Some factors to consider when pursuing this would be demonstrating that the molecular mechanisms recognised in all of these genomics research studies in primary lesions are also pertinent in the metastatic and recurrent settings, as drug development is generally decided to focus on tackling recurrent and metastasis disease. Second, parallel research of relevant biomarkers that could detect potential patient subsets receptive to present treatments should be prioritised. In addition to the currently available data on OSCC, the capacity to use genomics to predict drug responses, as well as the introduction of precise gene editing technologies, presents promising potential in the search of quality treatment modalities for OSCC patients [21].

3. Cancer genomics research potentials

Although large-scale research investigations have found a huge number of genetic changes that support the development and evolution of several types of cancer, some tumour types remain poorly understood. Many tumours could benefit from new technology and knowledge gathered from prior genomic research to characterise the full collection of genetic alterations and many other DNA and RNA changes. Researchers can find genomic abnormalities that may promote cancer by comparing genomic information from malignancies and normal tissue from same patient [22].

Another possibility is to broaden the existing use of genomic technologies to study the molecular basis of clinical characteristics. For example, this method could aid researchers in identifying genetic variations that distinguish aggressive malignancies

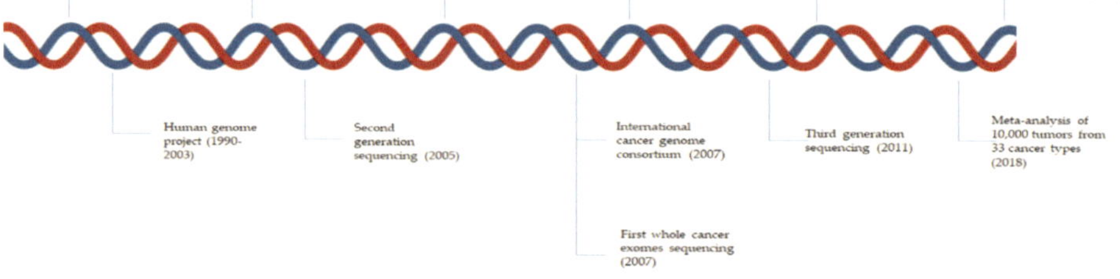

Figure 2.
In the previous 50 years, there have been significant developments in sequencing technology, seminal milestones, and large-cohort investigations modified.

from indolent cancers. Similar methodologies could be utilised to investigate the molecular mechanism of therapeutic response as well as treatment resistance mechanisms.

Patients' medical history and clinical data will increasingly be combined with the amount of data generated by cancer genomic studies. These combined findings could be utilised to generate more personalised cancer diagnosis and treatment techniques, as well as better methods for forecasting cancer risk, prognosis, and treatment response (**Figure 2**) [23].

4. Challenges in cancer genomics research

Comprehensive analyses of cancer genomes have revealed a wide range of genetic aberrations within tumours of the same type. Furthermore, only a small minority of these cancers are affected by recurrent genetic changes. Identifying which genetic variations cause cancer and uncovering unusual genetic mutations that cause cancer are thus difficult tasks for the research.

Another problem is obtaining high-quality biological samples for genetic investigations, which is especially difficult for tumour forms that are infrequent or rare, or those that are not treated predominantly with surgery.

Requirements involve establishing cell lines and animal studies that reflect the spectrum of human cancer. Many recurrent genetic lesions in human cancer have no models, and models for rare different types of cancer may be nonexistent or under represented.

Additional hurdles for the profession include managing and analysing the massive amounts of data generated by genetic investigations. This field of study necessitates a strong bioinformatics infrastructure and progressively relies on data and skills from multidisciplinary teams [24].

Author details

Sivapatham Sundaresan* and Lavanya Selvaraj
Department of Medical Research, SRM Medical College Hospital and Research Centre, SRM Institute of Science and Technology, Kattankalathur, Tamil Nadu, India

*Address all correspondence to: ssunsrm@gmail.com

References

[1] Zini A, Czerninski R, Sgan-Cohen HD. Oral cancer over four decades: Epidemiology, trends, histology, and survival by anatomical sites. Journal of Oral Pathology & Medicine. 2010;**39**(4):299-305

[2] Weisburger JH. Antimutagens, anticarcinogens, and effective worldwide cancer prevention. Journal of Environmental Pathology, Toxicology and Oncology: Official Organ of the International Society for Environmental Toxicology and Cancer. 1999;**18**(2):85-93

[3] Ferlay J, Shin HR, Bray F, Forman D, Mathers C, Parkin DM. Estimates of worldwide burden of cancer in 2008: GLOBOCAN 2008. International Journal of Cancer. 2010;**127**(12):2893-2917

[4] Khandekar SP, Bagdey PS, Tiwari RR. Oral cancer and some epidemiological factors: A hospital based study. Indian Journal of Community Medicine. 2006;**31**(3):157-159

[5] Nair DR, Pruthy R, Pawar U, Chaturvedi P. Oral cancer: Premalignant conditions and screening-an update. Journal of Cancer Research and Therapeutics. 2012;**8**(6):57

[6] Soames JV, Southam JC. Disorders of Development of Teeth and Craniofacial Anomalies. Oral Pathology. Oxford: Oxford University Press; 2005. pp. 3-17

[7] Graveland AP, Bremmer JF, De Maaker M, Brink A, Cobussen P, Zwart M, et al. Molecular screening of oral precancer. Oral Oncology. 2013;**49**(12):1129-1135

[8] Neville BW, Damm D, Allen C, Bouquot J. Oral and Maxillofacial Pathology, Ch. 14. St. Louis, Missouri: Saunders Elsevier; 2009. pp. 653-655

[9] Jerjes W, Upile T, Petrie A, Riskalla A, Hamdoon Z, Vourvachis M, et al. Clinicopathological parameters, recurrence, locoregional and distant metastasis in 115 T1-T2 oral squamous cell carcinoma patients. Head & Neck Oncology. 2010;**2**(1):1-21

[10] Okuyemi OT, Piccirillo JF, Spitznagel E. TNM staging compared with a new clinicopathological model in predicting oral tongue squamous cell carcinoma survival. Head & Neck. 2014;**36**(10):1481-1489

[11] Mardis ER. Next-generation DNA sequencing methods. Annual Review of Genomics and Human Genetics. 2008;**9**:387-402

[12] Choi M, Scholl UI, Ji W, Liu T, Tikhonova IR, Zumbo P, et al. Genetic diagnosis by whole exome capture and massively parallel DNA sequencing. Proceedings of the National Academy of Sciences. 2009;**106**(45):19096-19101

[13] Lechner M, Frampton GM, Fenton T, Feber A, Palmer G, Jay A, et al. Targeted next-generation sequencing of head and neck squamous cell carcinoma identifies novel genetic alterations in HPV+ and HPV-tumors. Genome Medicine. 2013;**5**(5):1-2

[14] Stransky N, Egloff AM, Tward AD, Kostic AD, Cibulskis K, Sivachenko A, et al. The mutational landscape of head and neck squamous cell carcinoma. Science. 2011;**333**(6046):1157-1160

[15] Agrawal N, Jiao Y, Bettegowda C, Hutfless SM, Wang Y, David S, et al. Comparative genomic analysis of esophageal adenocarcinoma and squamous cell carcinoma. Cancer Discovery. 2012;**2**(10):899-905

[16] Conesa A, Madrigal P, Tarazona S, Gomez-Cabrero D, Cervera A, McPherson A, et al. A survey of best practices for RNA-seq data analysis. Genome Biology. 2016;**17**(1):1-9

[17] Byron SA, Van Keuren-Jensen KR, Engelthaler DM, Carpten JD, Craig DW. Translating RNA sequencing into clinical diagnostics: Opportunities and challenges. Nature Reviews Genetics. 2016;**17**(5):257-271

[18] Costa V, Angelini C, De Feis I, Ciccodicola A. Uncovering the complexity of transcriptomes with RNA-Seq. Journal of Biomedicine and Biotechnology. 2010;**2010**:1-19

[19] Tang F, Barbacioru C, Wang Y, Nordman E, Lee C, Xu N, et al. mRNA-Seq whole-transcriptome analysis of a single cell. Nature Methods. 2009;**6**(5):377-382

[20] Marthong L, Ghosh S, Palodhi A, Imran M, Shunyu NB, Maitra A, et al. Whole genome DNA methylation and gene expression profiling of oropharyngeal cancer patients in north-eastern India: Identification of Epigenetically Altered Gene Expression Reveals Potential Biomarkers. Frontiers in Genetics. 2020;**11**(986):1-13

[21] Chai AW, Lim KP, Cheong SC. Translational genomics and recent advances in oral squamous cell carcinoma. In: Seminars in Cancer Biology. Vol. 61. Academic Press; 2020. pp. 71-83. DOI: 10.1016/j.semcancer.2019.09.011

[22] https://www.genengnews.com/topics/omics/genome-study-overhauls-cancer-categories-shifts-from-tissues-to-molecular-subtypes/

[23] Giunta S. Decoding human cancer with whole genome sequencing: A review of PCAWG project studies published in February 2020. Cancer and Metastasis Reviews. 2021;**40**(3):909-924

[24] https://www.cancer.gov/research/areas/genomics

Chapter 5

Dermatoscopy: A New Diagnostic Approach for Lesions on Mucous Membrane

Sahana Ashok

Abstract

Dermatoscope is used to examine the skin lesions without obstruction and is known as dermatoscopy or epiluminescence microscopy. Similarly, dermatoscope can be used to examine lesions on the mucous membrane of oral cavity. This is termed as "mucoscopy". Mucoscopy is an important upcoming digital tool for oral mucosal disorders. It can help to distinguish between the benign and malignant lesions, but needs to be correlated with clinical and histopathology if required. As literature on mucoscopy is minimal and is limited to individual case or case series. An organized, systemic analysis is very much essential on this topic. This chapter would focus on mucoscopic features of certain oral lesions which would help with further development and improvement of a non-invasive technique for diagnosis.

Keywords: mucoscopy, dermatoscopy, oral mucosa, lips, tongue

1. Introduction

Skin surface microscopy was introduced in 1663. Later a German dermatologist named Johann Saphier, added a light source as an improvisation to the device. The word "Dermoscopy" was coined first by a dermatologist named Goldman. Further, many universities, along with physicians and device manufacturing companies invented and patented many additions to the basic instrument [1, 2].

Dermatoscopy is a non-invasive and in vivo technique to appraise the pigmented skin lesions with a hand-held instrument or device termed as dermatoscope. However, it can also be used to examine lesions with little or no pigmentation [3]. The synonyms for this technique are Dermoscopy, epiluminescence microscopy, incident light microscopy, and skin-surface microscopy [4].

A dermatoscope is composed of an illuminating light source and a magnifying lens. The light source here can be nonpolarized or polarized. Polarized and nonpolarized light is combined with the magnifying lens and can be used as a surface contact or non-contact device [5, 6]. With this permutation and combination there are four types of dermatoscopes, they are

a. Polarized light, contact

b. Polarized light, non-contact

c. Non-polarized light, contact

d. Non-polarized light, non-contact

This device magnifies the structures or details that are not visible to the naked eye in the sub-dermal region of the epidermis, by 10 times for easy visualization. This magnification increases up to 70–80 times with a video recorder. Specialized add-ons like FotoFinder device (magnification up to 140×), camera attachments (magnification up to 400×) are available along with dermatoscope to capture images or recordings for storage or serial analysis [5, 7].

When dermatoscope is used to assess the mucosal surface is termed as 'mucoscopy'. However, the literature on mucoscopy is limited. Though observation of mucous membranes should be part of a dermatological examination usage of this device in mucoscopy is negligible. However, recent studies have shown that the potential of this instrument in mucoscopy. The aim of this chapter was to summarize the use of this device on mucous membrane [8].

2. Basic science of dermatoscope

When we use a device, knowing the science behind its working is of prime importance. Normally when a visible light falls on an object, it is either reflected, scattered, or absorbed by the object itself. If we consider skin as the object on which light falls, most of the light is reflected due to the increased refractive index of the stratum corneum (1.55) when compared with refractive index of air (1.0). Reflection from skin surface can be reduced by fixing a glass plate with refractive index 1.52 **Figure 1** and using an immersion fluid as an interface or by using polarizing filters **Figure 2** [9, 10].

Numerous immersion fluids like alcohols, water, oils and gels have been used. Most commonly used immersion medium being the alcohol (ethanol 70%) due to its low viscosity, amphiphilic solubility, disinfectant capability and image clarity. But in mucoscopy water soluble gels are preferred over alcohol because of their non-caustic property and higher viscosity [11]. Air bubbles along the immersion medium can hinder the clarity of structures under examination, because it creates a skin-air interface. It is very important to remove all the air bubbles before examination.

Another method to reduce the reflection from the assessing surface is by using polarizing light. In polarized light dermatoscope two filters are placed perpendicularly. When it reaches the surface of skin/mucous membrane, part of polarized light is scattered from surface and other part is scattered from deeper layers. The light reflected from surface causes glare, therefore is blocked by one of the attached filters. The light reflected by deeper layers is backscattered and makes it visible to the eye. This technique, which allows the light which has lost its polarization to pass through the second filter with additional blocking of the reflected light which maintains its polarization is known as "cross-polarization" [10, 12].

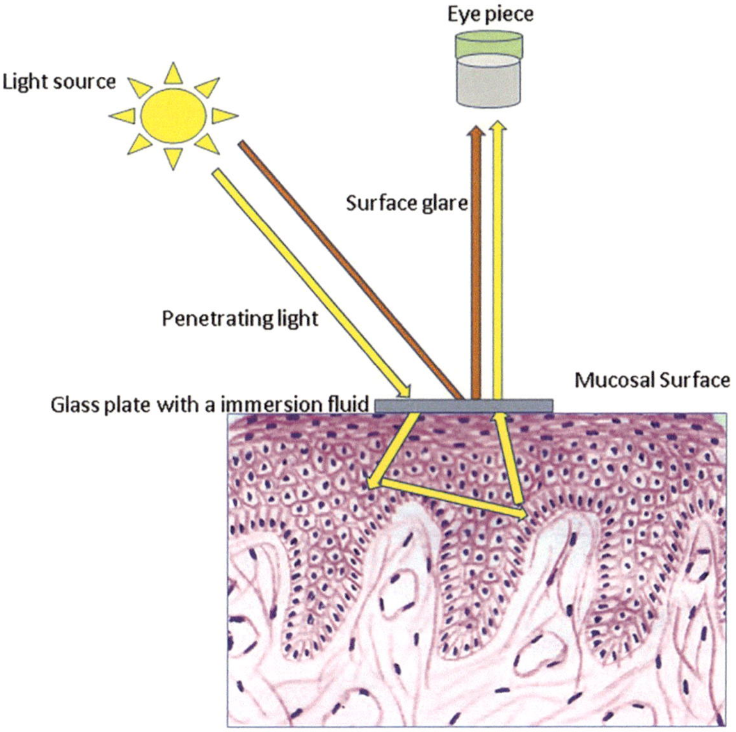

Figure 1.
Shows the working of a dermoscope using a glassplate with an immersion fluid.

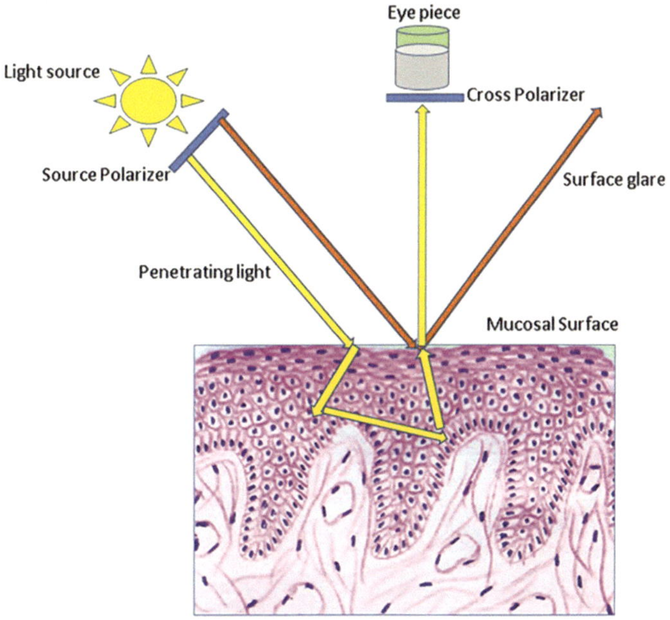

Figure 2.
Shows the working of a dermoscope using cross polarization.

2.1 Language of dermatoscopy

To acquire complete knowledge for using dermatoscopy on mucous membrane we need learn certain basic elements in this field. These elements are very important to describe and diagnose a skin/mucous lesions [13, 14].

A list of basic elements is as follows, **Figure 3**:

a. Lines (these straight objects present on the lesions which are longer in length than its width)

b. Globules (irregular objects with definite size and shape, easily identifiable due to its large size)

c. Pseudopod (one sided Dumble shaped)

d. Dots (shape is similar to globules, but are smaller in size)

e. Circles (ring like margin, which has a same center)

f. Structureless areas or blotches (any pattern of area which do not contain any definable above described objects)

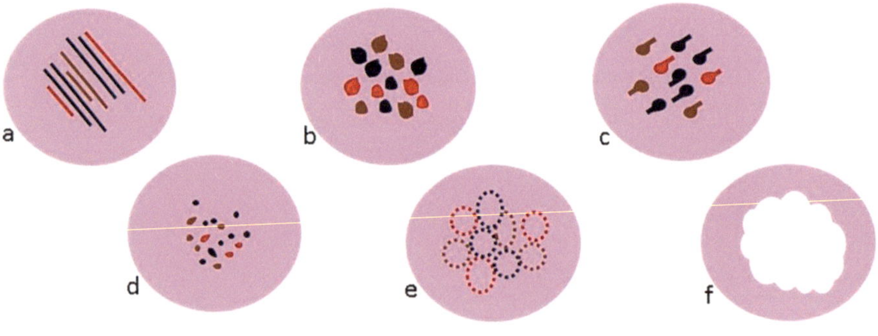

Figure 3.
Schematic diagram showing the basic elements of dermatoscopy.

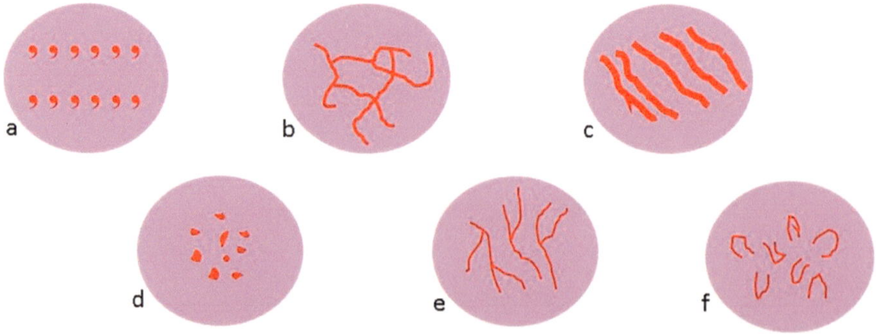

Figure 4.
Schematic diagram describing the vascular components seen in dermatoscopy.

There are certain terminologies used to describe a vascular component of a lesion, **Figure 4** [15].

a. Comma-shaped vessels

b. Perifollicular network of vessels

c. Dilated linear vessels

d. Doted blood vessels

e. Linear branching

f. Linear vessels with loops at their ends (hairpin vessels)

Other than these basic elements dermatoscopic lesions are evaluated on colors and harmony. Colors recognized are black, dark brown, orange, pink, white, gray, steel blue, purple, red and yellow [16]. With the knowledge of these basic elements of dermatoscopy we move ahead to describe known mucoscopic features of oral lesions.

3. Description of mucoscopic features of oral lesions

3.1 Fordyce's spots

These can be seen in any part of the oral mucosa due to presence of ectopic sebaceous glands. Mucoscopy shows whitish to yellowish separate round to oval structures corresponding to sebaceous glands with central opaque globules with small openings. These are surrounded by linear branched vessels [17].

3.2 Lingual varicosities

The sublingual veins in which there is degeneration of proteins in their elastic tissues are called as lingual varicosities. This is seen most frequently on the ventral surface of tongue. Mucoscopic features can be described as linear distribution of dark blue to black dilated vessels along with white shiny blotched areas [18].

3.3 Mucocele

This is the most common salivary gland cyst. It presents in two types based on the collection of mucus. Due to trauma if the salivary gland duct is severed and mucus collects in the connective tissue, then it is called extravasated type of mucocele. If the mucus is collected within the duct due its obstruction, then it is named as retention type of mucocele [19]. Mucoscopic features for this cyst is described in three different types [20].

Type I (retention/extravasated mucocele): purple in color and branched network of vessels.

Type II (due to recurrent trauma mucocele is associated surface hyperkeratosis): hyperkeratotic white areas with small unclear looped vessels.

Type III (lack of mucin material, healing stage): red in color, with yellowish areas and clear linear vessels with looped ends (hairpin vessels) [21].

3.4 Lichen planus

Lichen planus is considered as one of the potentially malignant disorders and a common mucocutaneous disease. In most of the lichen planus cases, oral lesions help in the early diagnosis of this disease, as they precede the skin lesions. Lichen planus has different clinical appearances and are described as—radiating white to gray, velvety, reticular patches, rings or streaks, thread-like or lacy papules in linear, annular or reticular forms [19]. Generally, symmetrical skin lesion is considered to be benign and asymmetrical as malignant. Sometimes odd shaped or irregular shaped lesions can also be benign. This holds good for mucosal lesions too [16]. Mucoscopy shows white reticular lines over a pink to purplish background. Sometimes crusts or scaling might also be seen in lip lesions. Tongue lesions display more curved vessels along with the above features. Dark skinned patients present a tricolored background (white + brown + red). Tiny erosions, globules, dots and mixed vascular pattern can be additional features depending on their clinical presentations [22].

3.5 Granular cell tumor

This is a benign tumor of neural origin (schwann cells). This tumor can be seen in any part of the body and in any age group, but more than half of the cases is seen in the oral cavity. Among the cases presenting in the oral cavity, more than one third are seen on lingual dorsum [19]. Yellowish to white structureless areas with surrounding polymorphic vessels are seen in mucoscopy, but the data are scant [23].

3.6 Pyogenic granuloma

This originates as a response of the tissues to nonspecific infections, therefore it's considered as reactive lesion. Three structures are mainly seen in the mucoscopy of these lesions—white linear lines representing the intra lobular fibrous septa, red homogenous areas and white area in a collar like fashion corresponding to hyperplastic epithelium [24, 25].

3.7 Haemangiomas and vascular malformations

Haemangiomas are tumors characterized by rapid endothelial cell proliferation, whereas vascular malformations results from anomalous development of vascular plexuses with normal endothelial cell growth cycle. Mucoscopic pattern of haemangiomas showed red pseudopods with network of white lines. Vascular malformations show thick elongated linear red or brownish lines in contrast to haemangiomas [26].

3.8 Anomalies of tongue

3.8.1 Black hairy tongue

The basic defect in hairy tongue is hypertrophy of filiform papillae. Typically, they are 1 mm in size, while filiform papillae in hairy tongue are greater than 10–15 mm in size. Generally, the condition is referred as black hairy tongue, however, the color may vary (brown, white, green or pink) depending on the etiology and secondary factors [19]. Mucoscopic features show brownish hairlike elongation of filiform papillae which are interspersed with white fungiform papillae [17].

3.8.2 Benign migratory glossitis

It is a psoriasiform mucositis with a characteristic feature of constantly changing pattern of white serpentine lines and surrounding areas of smooth and depapillated mucosa [27]. Under mucoscopy, reddish areas due to atrophy of filiform papillae and white lines demarcating the unchanged areas are seen [28].

3.8.3 Median rhomboid glossitis

This is a developmental anomaly of tongue because it is seen due to defective midline fusion of two lingual swellings and posterior fusion of tuberculum impar, leaving a rhomboid shaped smooth erythematous area. Features under mucoscopy shows desquamated or absence of lingual papillae and periphery of the lesion shows presence of normal papillae [28].

3.9 Aphthous stomatitis

This is a very common multifactorial disease with solitary or multiple painful ulcerations. Clinically these ulcers with gray membrane, necrotic centre and raised margins surrounded by erythematous halo [27]. Mucoscopically, yellowish to red central part encircled by a whitish structureless region and a circular edge of erythema [4].

3.10 Irritational fibroma

It is formed by the focal hyperplasia of connective tissue as a reaction to the induced trauma or irritation in the oral cavity. Dotted and irregular vessels are seen on a pinkish colored background under mucoscopy [29].

3.11 Pigmented lesions

The common pigmented lesions on oral mucosa are labial pigmented/melanotic macule, mucosal melanosis and physiological gingival melanin hyperpigmentation. Mucoscopic features of pigmented melanotic macule are reticular or parallel linear lines (including hyphal or fish-scale variants), dots or globules on surface, structureless area. In case of ephelides seen in Peutz-Jeghers or Addison disease we notice brownish, intertwined network "moth-eaten" borders or thick reticular lines with grayish granules or globules [30–32]. In case physiologic pigmented gingiva the mucosopic features is simply a homogenous brownish structureless area [33].

Amalgam tattoo is also one of the common pigmentations seen in the oral cavity. These pigmentations are seen as radio-opaque areas on radiographs [34], but mucoscopy shows structureless, homogenous, grainy, bluish pattern [35].

Oral melanoacanthoma also present as brown/black well-circumscribed macules or papules which may increase in size up to few centimeters [36]. Their starburst pattern with symmetric pigmented streaks along the lesion's periphery under mucoscopy can differentiate them from Peutz-Jeghers or Addison disease [35].

Melanocytic nevi are well defined macules. They can be congenital or acquired. They are classified as junctional, compound and intradermal/intramucosal. Mucoscopy of these macules show structurally homogeneous with wide or noticeable pigment network and streaks [34].

3.12 Cheilitis

It is a multifactorial disease affecting the lips. Due to varied aetiological factors the clinical presentation also varies, similarly the features under mucoscopy. Lesions associated with ulcerations presented with yellow to red structureless areas, fibrillar network. In allergic cheilitis yellowish to white scale and pinkish white structureless areas along with dotted vessels were evident. Few additional features to the later can be large red globules or scattered dotted vessels [37].

3.13 Squamous cell carcinoma

Squamous cell carcinoma (SCC) is the second most common malignancy. Even though the gold standard of diagnosis for squamous cell carcinoma is biopsy trailed by histopathological evaluation, non-invasive diagnostic tools have found increased attention. Dermoscopy has become one of the basic diagnostic methods in clinical practice. The most common dermoscopic features of non-invasive squamous cell carcinoma include clustered vascular pattern, glomerular vessels and hyperkeratosis [38]. Whereas invasive squamous cell carcinoma presents with a vascular polymorphism comprising of linear irregular, hairpin and grouped glomerular/dotted vessels over a whitish background with a central core of keratin or ulceration [39].

The clinic-dermoscopic-pathologic correlation can be shown with white-colored criteria, including scales/keratin, white circles, white halos and structureless whitish areas in well- or moderately differentiated variant. Whereas in poorly differentiated SCCs predominantly red color is seen which results from the presence of bleeding and/or dense vascularity, in the absence of scaling and keratin or other white-colored criteria. A diffuse distribution of vessels in various patterns and bleeding are signs of poor differentiation, while scaling is indicative of well- or moderately differentiated SCC [40]. Keratoacanthoma is a common low-grade tumor which closely resembles SCC microscopically. The most important dermoscopic features to keratoacanthoma and SCC are white circles, keratin crust/scale, blood spots, and white structurless zones. White circles are more common in SCC and keratin crust/scale in keratoacanthoma [38].

4. Conclusion

The dermatoscope has gained incredible popularity among dermatologists as an adjunctive tool to better visualize subsurface structures and identify patterns that may improve the diagnosis of a wide range of skin diseases. Similarly, mucoscopy should also be developed by analyzing many more cases on each above stated entities to confirm and support the findings. Difficulties in mucoscopy like hard-to-reach areas, contamination of instrument, conditions in which mouth opening difficulty is seen and cost effectiveness have to be encountered. The future of dermatoscopy/mucoscopy will involve combination of artificial intelligence that will make the assessment process increasingly objective, more accurate, and universally available. Despite the use of use dermatoscopy long, its widespread use on mucous membrane still remains unclear, whether it has decreased biopsy rates of benign lesions, reduced health care costs, or improved patient outcomes.

Author details

Sahana Ashok
GSL Dental College and Hospital, Rajahmundry, India

*Address all correspondence to: sahanarrr@yahoo.com

References

[1] Stolz W. Skin surface microscopy. The Lancet. 1989;**334**(8667):864-865

[2] Fricke D, Denker E, Heratizadeh A, Werfel T, Wollweber M. Non-contact dermatoscopic device with full polarization control and liquid lens based autofocus function. Roth Applied Sciences. 2019;**9**(11):2177

[3] Ascierto PA, Palmieri G, Celentano E, Parasole R, Caraco C, Daponte A, et al. Sensitivity and specificity of epiluminescence microscopy: Evaluation on a sample of 2731 excised cutaneous pigmented lesions. British Journal of Dermatology. 2000;**142**(5):893-898

[4] Hossam D, Sadek A, Saied N. Dermoscopy: A literature review. Egyptian Dermatology Online Journal. 2015;**11**:1

[5] Argenziano G, Soyer HP. Dermoscopy of pigmented skin lesions: A valuable tool for early diagnosis of melanoma. Lancet Oncology. 2001;**2**(7):443-449

[6] Vestergaard ME, Macaskill P, Holt PE, Menzies SW. Dermoscopy compared with naked eye examination for the diagnosis of primary melanoma: A meta-analysis of studies performed in a clinical setting. The British Journal of Dermatology. 2008;**159**(3):669-676

[7] Kamińska-Winciorek G, Placek W. The most common mistakes on dermatoscopy of melanocytic lesions. Postepy Dermatology in Alergology. 2015;**32**(1):33-39

[8] Hajar-Serviansky T, Gutierrez-Mendoza D, Galvan IL, Lammoglia Ordiales L, Mosqueda-Taylor A, Hernandez-Cázares M, et al. A case of oral mucosal melanoma. Clinical and dermoscopic correlation. Journal of Dermatological Case Report. 2012;**6**(1):1-4

[9] Ankad BS, Smitha SV, Koti VR. Basic science of dermoscopy. Clinical Dermatological Review. 2020;**4**(2):69-73

[10] Nirmal B. Dermatoscopy: Physics and principles. Indian Journal of Dermatopathology and Diagnostic Dermatology. 2017;**4**:27-30

[11] Gewirtzman AJ, Saurat JH, Braun RP. An evaluation of dermoscopy fluids and application techniques. The British Journal of Dermatology. 2003;**149**(1):59-63

[12] Benvenuto-Andrade C, Dusza SW, Agero AL, Scope A, Rajadhyaksha M, Halpern AC, et al. Differences between polarized light dermoscopy and immersion contact dermoscopy for the evaluation of skin lesions. Archives of Dermatology. 2007;**143**:329-338

[13] Johr RH, Stolz W. Dermoscopy from A to Z. In: Johr RH, Stolz W, editors. Dermoscopy—An Illustrated Self-Assessment Guide. New York: McGraw Hill; 2010. pp. 1-26

[14] Kittler H, Rosendah CA, Tschandl P, editors. Pattern analysis-basic principles. In: Dermatoscopy—An Algorithmic Method Based on Pattern Analysis. Vienna: Facultas; 2011. pp. 49-113

[15] Bowling J, editor. Introduction to dermoscopy. In: Diagnostic Dermoscopy: The Illustrated Guide. West Sussex: Wiley-Blackwell; 2012. pp. 2-14

[16] Oakley A. Dermatoscopic features [Internet]. 2008. Available from: dermatoscopy/

Dermatoscopicfeatures%20_%20 DermNet%20NZ.html [Accessed: August 23, 2021]

[17] Jakhar D, Kaur I. Mucoscopy of Fordyce's spots on lips. Indian Dermatology Online Journal. 2019;**10**(4):498-499

[18] Jha AK, Zeeshan MD, Jha Amar AK. Mucoscopy in lingual varicosities. Dermatology Practical and Conceptual. 2018;**8**(1):54-55

[19] Rajendran R. Benign and malignant tumors of the oral cavity. In: Shafers Textbook of Oral Pathology. 6th ed. Chennai: Elsevier; 2009. pp. 80-203

[20] Ayhan E, Toprak SF, Kaya Ş, Akkaynak S. Dermoscopy of oral mucocele: Three types of extravasation mucoceles. Turkish Journal of Medical Sciences. 2020;**50**(1):96-102

[21] Kaur I, Jakhar D, Anand P. Mucoscopy of mucocele. Indian Dermatology Online Journal. 2019;**10**(3):358-359

[22] Sonthalia S, Varma S, Jha AK, Jakhar D, Kaliyadan F. Case report: Dermoscopic features of oral lichen planus—The evolution of mucoscopy. F1000Research. 2018;7:284

[23] Mejía H, Rubiano MFO, Osorio VLD, Gonzalez MI. S100 negative granular cell tumor of the oral cavity: Dermoscopy and surgical approach. Anais Brasileiros de Dermatologia. 2019;**94**(1):79-81

[24] Oiso N, Kawada A. Dermoscopy of pyogenic granuloma on the lip: The differing appearances of vascular structures with and without pressure. European Journal of Dermatology. 2011;**21**(3):441

[25] Kissou A, Hassam BE. Dermoscopy of pyogenic granuloma. The Pan African Medical Journal. 2017;**27**:110

[26] Wassef M, Blei F, Adams D, et al. Vascular anomalies classification: Recommendations from the International Society for the Study of Vascular Anomalies. Pediatrics. 2015;**136**(1):e203-e214

[27] Neville BW, Damm D, Allenc R, Bouquot JE. Allergies and immunological diseases. In: Oral and Maxillofacial Pathology. 3rd ed. Philadelphia, PA: WB Saunders; 2009. pp. 330-332

[28] Rogers RS, Bruce AJ. The tongue in clinical diagnosis. Journal of the European Academy of Dermatology and Venereology. 2004;**18**:254-259

[29] Jiang M, Bu W, Chen X, Gu H. A case of irritation fibroma. Advances in Dermatology and Allergology. 2019;**36**(1):125-126

[30] Maymone MBC, Greer RO, Burdine LK, et al. Benign oral mucosal lesions: Clinical and pathological findings. Journal of the American Academy of Dermatology. 2019;**81**(1):43-56

[31] Gómez-Martín I, Collgros H, Ferguson PM, et al. Diagnostic accuracy of pigmented labial macules by in vivo reflectance confocal microscopy and correlation among techniques. Journal of the American Academy of Dermatology. 2020;**S0190-9622**(20):1-10

[32] Kim GW, Shin K, You HS, et al. Dermoscopic "Landscape Painting Patterns" as a clue for labial melanotic macules: An analysis of 80 cases. Annals of Dermatology. 2018;**30**(3):331-334

[33] Blum A, Simionescu O, Argenziano G, et al. Dermoscopy of pigmented lesions of the mucosa and the mucocutaneous junction: Results of a multicenter study by the International Dermoscopy Society (IDS). Archives of Dermatology. 2011;**147**(10):1181-1187

[34] Tuthill RJ. Weedon's skin pathology. The American Journal of Surgical Pathology. 2011;**35**:159

[35] Rossiello L, Zalaudek I, Ferrara G, Docimo G, Giorgio CM, Argenziano G. Melanoacanthoma simulating pigmented spitz nevus: An unusual dermoscopy pitfall. Dermatologic Surgery. 2006;**32**:735-737

[36] Alawi F. Pigmented lesions of the oral cavity: An update. Dental Clinics of North America. 2013;**57**:699-710

[37] Ito T, Natsuga K, Tanimura S, et al. Dermoscopic features of plasma cell cheilitis and actinic cheilitis. Acta Dermato-Venereologica. 2014;**94**(5):593-594

[38] Warszawik-Hendzel O, Olszewska M, Maj M, et al. Non-invasive diagnostic techniques in the diagnosis of squamous cell carcinoma. Journal of Dermatological Case Reports. 2015;**4**:89-97

[39] Rosendahl C, Cameron A, Argenziano G, et al. Dermoscopy of squamous cell carcinoma and keratoacanthoma. Archives of Dermatology. 2012;**148**(12):1386-1392

[40] Lallas A, Pyne J, Kyrgidis A, et al. The clinical and dermoscopic features of invasive cutaneous squamous cell carcinoma depend on the histopathological grade of differentiation. The British Journal of Dermatology. 2015;**172**:1308-1315

Chapter 6

Squamous Cell Carcinoma of Head and Neck

Chanyoot Bandidwattanawong

Abstract

Squamous cell carcinoma of head and neck (SCCHN) is the most common cancer arising in the head and neck region. Smoking and heavy alcohol drinking are still the well-established causes of most cases worldwide; however, human papillomavirus (HPV) infection is the concerning cause in the Western world. The different pathogenesis, pathophysiology, and prognosis between HPV-driven and non-HPV SCCHN would lead to the different treatment approaches. Breakthroughs in radiation techniques, better organ-preserving surgical strategies, and multidisciplinary management modalities are the major reasons for the curability rate among patients with early and locally advanced SCCHN. Unfortunately, among patients with advanced, recurrent, or metastatic diseases, the treatment remains an area of need. Such patients usually die within a few years. The immune checkpoint inhibitors have been shown to provide astonishingly better survival, but only among a small and not definitely known proportion of patients. Investigating the more specific biomarkers predicting the treatment response and novel therapeutic options is warranted. In this review, we highlight the latest advances in pathophysiology, treatment, and the future direction of researches.

Keywords: squamous cell carcinoma of head and neck, human papillomavirus, smoking, systemic therapy, radiotherapy, immunotherapy, immune checkpoint inhibitors, biomarkers

1. Introduction

Squamous cell carcinoma of head and neck (SCCHN) is cancer arising from the squamous epithelium in the oral cavity, pharynx, and larynx. It is the most common cancer that develops in the head and neck. According to the Global Cancer Statistics 2020, approximately 750,000 new cases were estimated and nearly 360,000 cases died annually. The lip and oral cavity are the most common sites, while, in respective order, larynx, oropharynx, and hypopharynx are less common sites [1]. Men are significantly more likely to develop SCCHN than women with an incidence ratio around 2:1 to 4:1 [2]. The average age of diagnosis is 50–70 years [3]. Globally, the incidence of HNSCC has increased by 36.5% over the past decade [4]. The prevalence of SCCHN varies across regions of the world and has been presumably correlated with tobacco use, excessive alcohol consumption, or both. There has been a significant decline in tobacco uses in Western countries during the last few decades, which has led to a sharp decline in smoking-related SCCHN [5]. On the contrary, there has been a significant increase in global epidemics of human papillomavirus (HPV)-associated SCCHN [6–8]. Around one-eighth of the incident cases of SCCHN comprise oropharyngeal squamous cell carcinoma (OPSCC), with HPV being an important associated risk factor for its development. HPV infection would be implicated with a small number of other SCCHN subsites. Data in this regard are quite inconclusive, presumably as a result of insufficient details on anatomical tumor localization and different HPV detection methods [9]. SCCHN of the oral cavity, hypopharynx, and larynx are associated with smoking and are categorized into HPV-negative SCCHN. No screening strategy has proved to be effective, unfortunately. Vigilant and careful physical examination of the population at risk remains the effective approach for early detection [3, 4]. With the exception of early-stage carcinomas of lip and oral cavity which surgery is the main curative treatment (with radiotherapy or chemo-radiotherapy as the adjuvant treatment depending on disease stage and clinical risk or laryngeal cancers that are amenable to either surgery or radiotherapy/chemo-radiotherapy), the majority of patients with SCCHN need multi-modality approaches. In this review, the latest advances in the pathophysiology of both HPV and non-HPV-driven SCCHN and their impact on the management will be elucidated. Perspectives on future directions will be provided as well.

2. Epidemiology and pathophysiology of HNSCC

2.1 HPV-associated SCCHN

2.1.1 Pathophysiology

Human papillomavirus (HPV) has been recognized as the major cause of oropharyngeal squamous cell carcinoma (OPSCC). HPV is sexually-transmitted. Early sexual experience as well as a high number of sexual partners, especially oral sex partners, and previous genital warts are the risks for HPV-associated (HPV(+)) OPSCC. There is a higher prevalence of HPV(+) OPSCC in men compared with women, and white populations compared with Asians and black populations [10–12]. The prevalence varies from less than 10% of all OPSCC cases in developing countries to 60–70% in the United States [13–15]. These variabilities are supposed to be, at least in part, due to the difference in sensitivity and specificity of the HPV detection assays, characteristics of the study cohorts, and their confounded risk factors especially tobacco uses and alcohol consumptions in the study population [16]. HPV infects the stratified squamous epithelia, both cutaneous and mucosal including the skin of hands and feet, as well as the anogenital tract, mouth, throat, and respiratory tract. Tonsillar crypt cells, similar to uterine cervical squamocolumnar junction cells, are arranged in a discontinuous single-layered epithelium that is more susceptible to cellular transformation than cells within other parts of the head and neck region [17, 18]. These perplexed invaginated crypts are naturally designed to entrap bacteria and foreign materials, driving the expression of programmed cell death-1 ligand-1 (PD-L1) [13]. The PD- L1 is responsible for immune evasion by binding programmed death-1 (PD-1) receptors expressed by the immune cells; therefore, the PD-L1 overexpression in tonsils promotes persistent HPV infection allowing carcinogenesis [14]. Moreover, in tonsillar crypts, the establishment of a biofilm composed of bacterial microcolonies encased in a glycocalyx matrix contributes to the HPV capability to escape the immune system [15]. The HPV family composes of circular, double-stranded DNA viruses of 8000 base pairs encoding proteins involved in viral replication (E1 and E2/E4) and assembly (L1 and L2), as well as accessory proteins (E5, E6, and E7). High-risk HPV types, including HPV16, HPV18, HPV31, HPV33, HPV35, HPV39, HPV45, HPV51, HPV52, HPV56, HPV58, HPV59, and HPV68, can induce malignant transformation of the infected oropharyngeal epithelium [19] by disrupting cell-cycle check points through E6- and E7-mediated degradation of p53 and Rb proteins, respectively [20]. Furthermore, the integration of the viral genome leads to E6/E7 expression, followed by disruption of the E2 coding region and dysregulation of E6/E7 themselves. This enables HPV to create the condition of persistent infections and replications. While the infected epithelial cells are gradually differentiated, the viral proteins are synthesized; however, no viral particle is actually produced. This non-productive infection by HPV is a key for cancer formation [21]. During carcinogenesis, the HPV E6 and E7 oncoproteins decrease the levels of p53 and functional Rb by post-translational regulation, resulting in aberrant overexpression of the cell-cycle protein p16 [22], which can be detected by immunohistochemistry (IHC) [23], rationalizing its use as a surrogate marker for the emergence of high-risk HPV-inducing cancer transformation rather than the infection as detected by an HPV DNA assay. Nevertheless, p16 expression is frequently lost in most cancers due to gene mutations, deletions, or promoter methylation [24], and p16 silencing has been reported to be as a result of tobacco exposure [25], indicating that this marker should be used carefully in the co-presence of risk factors. Interestingly, alcohol consumption is also correlated with p16 loss [26]. Thus, in non-OPSCC patients (mostly HPV negative) other risk factors can affect p16 status.

2.1.2 Prognosis

HPV status classifies OPSCC in particular into two distinct diseases (HPV(+) and HPV(−)) and it is still the only clinically biomarker that has been extensively validated from both retrospective and prospective studies. Several studies have shown that patients with HPV(+) OPSCC, as identified through PCR, *in situ* hybridization, or p16 immunohistochemistry (IHC) on tumor tissues, have shown that HPV(+) tumors are more likely to present with earlier T stage (T1-T2) and well-defined borders [27] or even occult primary tumors but have higher N stage (usually cystic and involving multi-level of the cervical lymph nodes) [28], and usually have poorer tumor differentiation, either non-keratinizing or basaloid histopathology [27]. Furthermore, the studies on correlation with clinical and imaging characteristics revealed that it usually had well-defined contours with exophytic growth (less necrotic and less ulcerated) and trended to uninvolved muscle tissue [28, 29]. Smoking also influenced clinical and imaging manifestations of HPV(+) OPSCC that were different from HPV(+) OPSCC in non-smoker [29]. The incidence of distant metastases seemed to be lower and if occurred, metastases usually developed later and with a very different pattern from patients with HPV(−) one. HPV(+) OPSCC had a 28% reduction in the risk of death and a 49% reduction in the risk of disease recurrence [30]. Second, primary tumor in patients with HPV(+) OPSCC is uncommon, and more likely to have a better overall survival rate compared to patients with

HPV(−) ones [31]. The significantly better overall and disease-free survival compared with patients with HPV(−) have been confirmed by many prospective phase 3 clinical trials [30, 32–39]. Even after adjustment for differences in favorable prognostic factors that were usually associated with HPV-positive patients (younger age, better performance status, fewer co-morbidities, less-or never-smoking) [32]. Consequently, numerous studies agreed on the fact that HPV(+) OPSCC led to a survival difference of up to 26.9% over HPV(−) one [40]. Smoking, on the other hand, has a negative impact on treatment efficiency and survival outcome. Smoking blunted the positive impact of HPV on survival as well. HPV(+) non-smoker had better prognosis compared with HPV(+) smoker, regardless of HPV detection methods (HPV DNA PCR, ISH, p16 IHC) used [41]. Since HPV(+) differs from and has a more favorable prognosis than HPV(−) OPSCC, the recently released Eighth Edition of the American Joint Committee on Cancer proposed the staging algorithm specifically for HPV(+) OPSCC, distinguishing it from HPV negative OPSCC. According to the new staging system, 92% of patients with HPV-positive OPSCC could be downstage, and up to 64% of patients were now staged as stage I disease [42]. Van Gysen et al. conducted a retrospective cohort study to validate the new AJCC staging system for HPV(+) OPSCC and demonstrated that this system better discriminated between stage I and stage II HPV(+) OPSCC with respect to OS compared with the seventh edition staging system. However, further investigation was required for stage III or IV patients [43].

2.1.3 HPV detection strategies

HPV testing in OSCC varies in detection targets including HPV DNA polymerase chain reaction (PCR) for E6/E7 viral oncogenes, HPV E6/E7 mRNA detection quantitative reverse transcription-PCR (qRT-PCR), DNA *in situ* hybridization (ISH), RNA ISH, and p16 immunohistochemical staining (IHC) as a surrogate marker for HPV status [44]. There is still no consensus regarding which method should be the gold standard. The PCR techniques are complex and have low specificity because they cannot distinguish between HPV acting as an oncogenic driver and transcriptionally silent virus from non-pathogenic or contaminated one [45]. Even though the detection of viral E6/E7 mRNA by RT-PCR is widely accepted as the gold standard due to its higher sensitivity, more specificity in detection of the oncogenic viral mRNA/DNA target, and its feasibility on formalin-fixed, paraffin-embedded tissue (FFPE) block [46], there are serious limitations including its time-consuming and its decreasing sensitivity depending on the quality of samples. The DNA ISH is another molecular test with high specificity, which enables direct detection of the presence of oncogenic HPV in matched topographical relationship with pathological samples, ascertaining that the pathogenic viral DNA emerges from tumor cells and not surrounding normal tissues. Furthermore, ISH has the advantage of being feasible in both FFPE tissues; however, this technique still lacks sufficient clinical validation. The DNA ISH is currently not used in routine practice [47]. Lydiatt et al. suggested that the test should be simple, inexpensive, and reproducible [42]. Not only the p16 IHC is the well-established marker as a surrogate for the presence of the oncogenic HPV, but also an independent positive prognostic factor among patients with OPSCC [48]. In particular, the cutoff point for p16 overexpression is diffuse (more than 75%) tumor expression localized to tumor cell nuclei and cytoplasm, with at least moderate (2+ or 3+) staining intensity. Either cytoplasmic-only staining or staining on other non-oropharyngeal sites is considered non-specific [49].

2.2 HPV-negative (−) SCCHN

2.2.1 Pathophysiology

Tobacco smoking is classified as being carcinogenic to humans by the International Agency for Research on Cancer (IARC) [50] and there are strong supporting evidences of association with head and neck cancer [51]. The HPV(−) SCCHN is characteristically seen in patients with a history of heavy tobacco and alcohol use [52]. Interestingly, HPV(−) SCCHN can occur in relatively young patients without a history of tobacco use, and the incidence has been rising with unclarified etiology [53]. Different brands of cigarettes and cigars use varying formulations of blended tobaccos affecting the various amount of nicotine and carcinogen content, thus impacting the toxicity of the smoke [54]. Smokeless tobacco products such as chewing tobacco, snuff, gutkha, and betel quid have been associated with oral cavity cancer for several decades. Some of the added components to these products can promote or modulate the absorption rate of nicotine. Areca nut commonly used in chewing tobacco products in India and Southeast Asia contains the alkaloid drugs arecoline, muscarine, and pilocarpine, which cause cholinergic mood-relaxing effects promoting addictive effect [18]. The pH of a tobacco product affects the rate of nicotine absorption. Buffering substances such as slacked lime or calcium carbonate that usually consist in gutkha and betel quid result in elevating the pH; therefore, they enhance the rate of nicotine absorption [55]. Both tobacco and especially tobacco fume are loaded with polycyclic aromatic hydrocarbons (PAH) and nitrosamines, which are the established human carcinogens and are strongly related to the risk of SCCHN. Their reactive metabolites, if not appropriately detoxified and excreted, lead to DNA damage, characteristically by promoting the generation of bulky DNA adducts. If such damages are not accurately and promptly repaired, the permanent damages as demonstrated by mutations, deletions, and amplifications can emerge. The *TP53* and *CDKN2A* that encode p53 and $p16^{INK4A}$, respectively, are the most common genomic abnormalities in HPV(−) SCCHN. Furthermore, signaling pathways such as phosphoinositide 3-kinase (PI3K)–AKT–mTOR and MAPK pathway genes are mutagenically overactivated. Such genetic abnormalities are associated with the onset, progression, and adverse prognosis of HPV-negative SCCHN [56]. The fact that *TP53* mutations in SCCHN have distinct signatures from *TP53* mutations with aging and ultraviolet light exposure indicates the truly different mechanisms of genetic damage [57]. In contrast to HPV(+) OPSCC that the *TP53* gene is rarely altered, since p53 in HPV(+) OPSCC is eliminated by the action of E6 [56]. Excessive alcohol drinking is known to synergize with tobacco use to promote the carcinogenesis of HPV(−) SCCHN, in particular. It is postulated that alcohol would function as a solvent for carcinogens to enhance the exposure of epithelial cells to these substances [58]. Alcohol is metabolized to acetaldehyde inducing the DNA adducts [59].

2.2.2 Prognosis

One of the unique characteristics of tobacco smoking-induced squamous cell carcinoma is the development of synchronous and/or metachronous second primary tumors arising at an exceptionally high rate after the diagnosis of an initial primary tumor and can be occurred along the aero-digestive tract including the head and neck, esophagus, and lungs [60]. The concept of "field cancerization" suggests that the carcinogens trigger the genomic damages along with the large anatomical fields as far as the tobacco fume can approach [61]. There are evidences supporting that the size of the damaged anatomical field may increase with patient age, as well [62]. A pooled analysis within the International Head and Neck Epidemiology Consortium demonstrated that besides older ages at diagnosis and advanced tumor staging that were the consistent adverse prognostic factors of survival, cigarette smoking was an independent unfavorable prognostic factor for overall survival (OS) among patients with OPSCC. Intense smoking (as defined as >20 cigarettes/day) was also an independent prognostic factor for OS among patients with oral cavity cancer. On the contrary, among patients with laryngeal cancer, low educational level was rather a deleterious prognostic factor for OS; moreover, the intensity of alcohol drinking was the prognostic factor for both of the OS and head-and-neck-cancer-specific survival [63].

Apart from the carcinogenic effects of tobacco, abundant evidence have demonstrated adverse effects of tobacco on various treatment-related outcomes in patients with SCCHN, including radiotherapy efficacy, surgical outcomes, and wound complications. Chen et al. reported that continued smoking during receiving radiotherapy was associated with inferior 5-year overall survival, locoregional control, and disease-free survival [64]. In addition, patients undergoing surgical treatment for SCCHN who were current or former smokers were more likely to have various postoperative complications including wounds and infections resulting in a longer length of stay than never smokers [65]. Marin et al. conducted a prospective study on the effect of smoking on wound healing in smokers undergoing free tissue transfer and concluded that those who were current smokers as indicated by high serum cotinine concentration, a metabolite of nicotine, would predict an increased risk of wound complication [66].

3. Management of newly diagnosed, early, and locally advanced SCCHN

3.1 Primary surgical approaches in SCCHN

Primary surgical treatment is usually considered as the standard of care for oral-cavity cancers, carcinoma of the true glottis, and sino-nasal cancers. The oral cavity cancers (OCC) are easily accessible trans-orally. Both the true glottis larynx (vocal folds) and paranasal sinus are void of lymphatics. Therefore, the primary surgical approach is the treatment of choice for such cancers and is associated with high cure rates with acceptable morbidity. In the case of oral cavity cancers, it has been recognized that the prognosis of OCC worsens when the tumor is thicker. The revised AJCC 8th edition cancer staging manual emphasizes the significance of the depth of invasion (DOI). For every 5-mm increase in DOI (microscopically measured from the level of the basement membrane of the closest adjacent normal mucosa), both cT and pT categories are right now categorized to one level increasing according to the following: ≤ 5 mm, >5 mm but ≤10 mm, and > 10 mm [42]; therefore, the DOI should be taken into account prior to consideration of surgery with curative intent. Besides oral, laryngeal, and sino-nasal cancers, the primary surgical approach is more suitable for stage I-II diseases. Oropharyngeal cancers (OPC) may be managed by either primary surgery or radiotherapy with the comparable outcomes [67, 68].

Among patients with laryngeal cancer, definitive chemoradiotherapy (CRT) is the time-honored preferred treatment, especially for the reason of organ preservation. Surgery is usually reserved as salvage treatment. According to the landmark RTOG

91–11, local control and larynx-preservation rates were significantly higher with concomitant cisplatin and RT (definitive CCRT); however, the OS curves separated after 4 years, favoring induction chemotherapy (IC) followed by RT alone. Although CCRT had the lowest rates of cancer-related deaths, it also had the highest rate of non-cancer deaths compared with IC, presumably attributed to late swallowing dysfunction and aspiration [69]. Patel et al. conducted a real-world retrospective analysis of treatment outcomes between surgical (partial laryngectomy (PL) or total laryngectomy (TL) with or without adjuvant radiotherapy with or without concomitant chemotherapy) and non-surgical (definitive CCRT)) management among 8703 patients with non-T1, stage III/IV, glottic, and supraglottic cancer from the National Cancer Data Base during 2003–2011. They demonstrated that non-surgical definitive CRT resulted in equivalent survival outcomes among patients with non-T4, low nodal burden (N0-N1) disease, and even better than surgical management (with or without adjuvant treatment) among patients with non-T4, high nodal burden (N2-N3) disease. However, patients with T4 disease, TL followed by adjuvant RT, or CCRT had superior survival outcomes compared with non-surgical definitive CCRT [70]. This study did not analyze the outcomes of IC, which was commonly used in the current practice of organ preservation. Also noted was the fact that not all T4 diseases were amenable to curative surgery especially those with T4b and those with supraglottic primary.

Since head and neck cancers have a propensity to metastasize to cervical lymph nodes, lymphatic drainage of the primary site and the risk of occult metastatic spread guide decisions regarding additional therapy. *Radical neck dissection (RND)* is to remove neck nodes of levels I–V, accessory nerve, internal jugular vein, and sternomastoid muscle, and this procedure is compulsory for most of the diseases with obviously clinical lymph node metastasis. If preservation of one or more of the accessory nerve, internal jugular vein, or sternomastoid muscle is possible, the procedure is called *modified radical neck dissection (MRND)* (types I, II, III, respectively). If removal of one or more additional lymphatic and/or non-lymphatic structures(s) relative to a RND, for example, level VII, retropharyngeal lymph nodes, hypoglossal nerve is necessary to eradicate all of the suspicious sites, it is called extended radical neck dissection (ERND). If the reservation of one or more levels of lymph nodes is possible, the procedure is called *selective node dissection (SND)*. SND is usually indicated for clinical node-negative disease with a higher chance of occult lymphatic metastasis, that is, when a primary tumor deeply invades (ipsilateral removal of the most possible lymph node groups with tumor spread) or when primary tumor at a site with rich lymphatics crosses the midline (contralateral removal) [71].

More recently, transoral robotic surgery (TORS) and transoral laser microsurgery (TLM) have emerged as the primary surgical modalities in the management of oropharyngeal carcinoma (OPSCC), in particular. As compared with standard open surgery, these techniques have been shown to reduce hospital stays and feeding tube requirements at 1 year [72]. In OPSCC, TORS is suitable for the management of small-sized tumors (cT1–T2) [73]. Even though, about 17–31% of patients who underwent TORS eventually needed to receive salvage radiotherapy and/or chemotherapy. Thus, about a quarter of these patients eventually needed multi-modality therapy.

3.2 Multi-modality approach in locally advanced SCCHN

More than 60% of patients present with stage III or IV disease, which is characterized by large tumors with extensive local invasion (clinical T3–4) and metastases to regional nodes, or both. Locally advanced disease is associated with a high risk of local recurrence (15 to 40%) and distant metastasis, with a grave prognosis (5-year OS, <50%) [74]. A dilemma usually exists between whether it would take to completely remove a bulky or extensively infiltrated tumor versus the impact such a resection would have on the patient's quality of life and self-image. When surgical resection is not feasible due to in-operable diseases, pre-existing serious co-morbidities, or on the condition that curative surgery would lead to unacceptable long-term functional and or cosmetic outcomes, the definitive concurrent chemo-radiotherapy (CCRT) is the most suitable choice.

The recent American Joint Commission on Cancer (AJCC) revised the T-staging classifications of head and neck cancers [42]. The T4 disease is subcategorized into T4a and T4b designations. Most patients with T4b tumors are generally defined as definitely unresectable, whereas the T4a tumors are potentially resectable. However, they need more devoted surgical techniques, if curative intent is primarily considered. The T4b is characterized by one of the following features: 1) vascular encasement and invasion, 2) prevertebral space invasion, and 3) invasion of mediastinal structures. The locally advanced disease generally harbors high-risk adverse features. The independent pathologic risk factors for recurrence include T3 or T4 tumors, multiple involved nodes, lymphovascular invasion, anatomic location, low neck location of lymph node involvement, extra-nodal extension (ENE), perineural invasion, and close/positive margins [75–77]. The more number of risk factors, the more the chance such a patient has increased risk of recurrence [78]. In addition, poorly differentiated tumors and, especially for oral cavity cancers, the depth of invasion (DOI) would be at risk for recurrence [79]. Consequently, all patients with stage III-IV diseases need postoperative radiotherapy (PORT) as a part of treatment with curative intent. Two large randomized controlled trials, the EORTC 22931 [80] and the RTOG 9501 [81], demonstrated a statistically significant loco-regional control (LRC) benefit with the addition of cisplatin of 100 mg/m^2 to PORT, given every 3 weeks for three cycles for patients with "high-risk" features. Both studies reported that serious (grade ≥ 3) toxicity occurred more than doubled with the addition of chemotherapy. However, the rate of distant metastasis did not differ between arms. When the results of the EORTC and RTOG trials were analyzed in a meta-analysis, a statistically significant OS improvement was determined in favor of postoperative adjuvant chemo-radiotherapy, especially for patients with ENE and close/positive surgical margins [82]. An OS benefit of an alternative schedule of cisplatin administration of weekly 50 mg/m^2 added to PORT was also demonstrated for stage III/IV SCCHN with ENE; however, the LRC was not proven [83]. The Japanese group (JCOG 1008) trial also showed the non-inferiority of the alternative schedule weekly cisplatin 40 mg/m^2 to three-weekly cisplatin in high-risk patients with microscopically positive margin and/or ENE [84]. In general, PORT should be commenced within 6 weeks after surgery [85]. A meta-analysis by Matuschek et al. showed no improvement in OS, PFS, or LRC with post-operative accelerated fractionation compared with conventional fractionation [86]; however, among patients with stage III/IV and a prolonged interval from surgery to RT, the accelerated fractionation seemed to result in better DFS or LRC benefit [87].

The recent MACH-NC meta-analysis revealed that chemotherapy when used concomitant with radiotherapy (RT) either as definitive treatment or following surgery in case of pathological adverse features led to an absolute benefit of 6.5% at 5 years and 3.6% at 10 years. Concomitant chemotherapy showed a significant effect on loco-regional failure (LRF), but not on distant failure (DF). For event-free survival (EFS), the meta-analysis demonstrated the highest effect for poly-chemotherapy with platin salt (HR = 0.74 [0.67; 0.82]) and the lowest for mono-chemotherapy without platin salt (0.86 [0.80, 0.93]). However, for OS, the interaction was borderline significant. Notable, the effect of chemotherapy on survival was decreasing with increasing age, probably due to the fact that more non-cancer deaths were reported more among patients 70 or over. The induction chemotherapy (IC), on the other hand, did not improve the LRF rate, OS, and EFS, even though it could decrease DF. There was no significant variation of the effect on OS according to the type of induction chemotherapy. The docetaxel/cisplatin/5-FU (TPF) regimen seemed to perform best in terms of EFS, but not OS compared with other regimens. Neither OS nor EFS was improved with adjuvant chemotherapy (AC). Moreover, AC led to a significant decrease in LRF and DF, as well as the deleterious effect on 120-day mortality [88]. Gau et al. suggested that IC (TPF regimen, in particular) might have less interest in OPSCC, especially among those associated with HPV. The IC would be most preferential if functional laryngeal preservation is the priority [89]. Petit et al. performed an individual patient data network meta-analysis to compare various kinds of multimodality management with loco-regional therapy alone (surgery, RT, or both) in patients with locally advanced SCCHN. Hyper-fractionated RT with CCRT (HFCRT) was ranked as the best treatment for OS, whereas IC with TPF regimen followed by locoregional therapy ($IC_{Tax\text{-}PF}$-LRT), accelerated RT with CCRT (ACRT), IC with TPF regimen followed by concomitant chemo-radiotherapy (IC_{TaxPF}-CLRT) and CCRT with platinum-based chemotherapy ($CLRT_P$) were ranked less in consecutive order. Unfortunately, the treatment-related toxicities were not included in the analysis, even though HFCRT would be too toxic to be assigned in routine practice [90].

Among patient's ineligible to cisplatin, either carboplatin/5-FU or carboplatin/paclitaxel are both the acceptable alternatives used in concomitant with RT [67].

3.3 De-escalation strategy for HPV-associated OPSCC

Since HPV(+) OPSCC is characteristically more radio-sensitive and chemo-sensitive than cancers caused by smoking and alcohol, the conventional paradigms like postoperative RT involving both tumor bed and neck with or without concomitant chemotherapy or definitive high-dose of RT in concomitant with high-dose cisplatin seem to be too toxic without incremental survival benefits. De-escalation of therapy has been proposed for this particular sub-group based on data demonstrating high OS and PFS [91]. De-escalation strategy includes minimally-invasive surgery, reduced dose and target volumes of adjuvant RT, and potential omission of chemotherapy.

Transoral robotic surgery (TORS) is a minimally invasive approach that reduces morbidity compared with traditional, open surgery most suitable for patients with resectable tonsil or base of tongue tumors when the adequate functional outcome can be preserved. The ORATOR2 study is an ongoing randomized trial investigating de-escalated definitive RT-based treatment in comparison with surgery with de-escalated adjuvant therapy. Both survival and swallowing quality of life will be evaluated [92].

ECOG-ACRIN 3311 was a randomized trial investigating reduced dose adjuvant RT for patients with intermediate postoperative risk factors. Patients with "low-risk" (AJCC 7th ed. pT1-T2, N0–1) disease with negative margins were observed, while patients with "intermediate risk" (close margins, < 1 mm of ENE, 2 to 4 involved lymph nodes, perineural invasion, or lymphovascular invasion) were randomized to postoperative RT of either 50 or 60 Gy. "High-risk" (positive margins, > 1 mm of ENE, or ≥ 5 involved nodes) patients received standard concurrent RT with cisplatin. At a median follow-up of 35.1 months, the outcomes were comparable or even better than historical results, and the 3-year PFS rates were 96.9%, 94.9%, 93.5%, and 90.7%

for the low-risk, 50 Gy, 60 Gy, and high-risk arms, respectively [93]. The PATHOS trial is an ongoing randomized trial investigating a reduction in adjuvant RT and chemotherapy. Patients with low-risk disease are observed postoperatively, patients with intermediate-risk factors are randomized to 50 Gy vs. 60 Gy, and patients with high-risk features are randomized to 60 Gy alone or 60 Gy with cisplatin [94].

Omission of chemotherapy was studied in the randomized phase 2 NRG-HN002 trial. Patients with p16-positive, AJCC 7th ed. T1-T2 N1-N2b or T3 N0-N2b OPSCC with 10 or fewer pack-years of smoking were randomized to the "standard-of-care," 60 Gy of RT in 6 weeks with cisplatin vs. 60 Gy of RT in 5 weeks without any systemic therapy. The 2-year PFS rate was 90.5% for cisplatin/RT vs. 87.6% for RT alone. Unfortunately, RT alone arm did not meet the prespecified 95% confidence interval threshold for PFS superiority to 85%; moreover, there was no difference in swallowing quality of life between the 2 arms [95].

Cetuximab, an epidermal growth factor receptor (EGFR) chimeric IgG1 monoclonal antibody, was shown to improve survival when used concurrently with RT in patients with locally advanced SCCHN as compared with RT alone leading to its popularity for use concurrently with RT as an alternative to cisplatin, especially among patients ineligible to cisplatin due to impaired renal function. Subgroup analysis showed superior survival benefit among patients with p16+. Cetuximab also had less nephrogenic (usually mild hypomagnesemia and hypokalemia) than cisplatin. Therefore, cetuximab had been investigated as a de-escalation strategy; however, three randomized phases 3 trials RTOG 1016 [96], De-ESCALaTE HPV [97], and TROG 12.01 [98] demonstrated the statistically significant detriment in both PFS and OS for patients treated with cetuximab/RT. In addition, toxicities were not overall reduced with cetuximab/RT compared with cisplatin/RT.

In conclusion, while results from well-designed clinical trials are gathering, the current data are still insufficient to recommend any de-intensified treatment strategy for HPV-associated OPSCC to be implemented in routine clinical practice.

3.4 Post-treatment response assessment and the role of salvage surgery

Since more than two-thirds of SCCHN patients present with locally advanced disease, usually not amenable to curative surgery, definitive chemo-radiotherapy is, therefore, the treatment of choice. Recurrence rates as high as 60% within 2 years of treatment have been reported with 20–30% of patients developing the distant metastatic disease [99]. Such patients mandate accurate staging and response assessment to guide appropriate management. Combined fluorine-18 fluorodeoxyglucose (F^{18}-DG) positron emission tomography-computed tomography (PET-CT) is capable of both determining extent of locoregional and distant disease at initial staging and assessment post-treatment response [100]. Data from randomized controlled trials have shown that PET-CT is a precise and cost-effective technique for assessing response and would lead to spare 80% of patients from unnecessary salvage neck dissection [101]. Nevertheless, post-treatment-related changes in the neck can make assessment problematic in some cases, due to evidence suggesting that HPV(+) OPSCC may behave differently to HPV(−) SCCHN [102]. The semi-quantitative methods of treatment response assessment using standardized uptake value (SUV) alone have not been shown to be accurate at assisting a physician's decision. The more reproducible qualitative interpretative criteria have been developed and validated in clinical trials to determine their value in predicting residual loco-regional disease and would help limit the number of problematically equivocal scan results [103–105].

Zhong et al. conducted a clinical trial to compare the accuracy of four different qualitative interpretative criteria (NI-RADS, Porceddu, Hopkins, Deauville) for predicting loco-regional control and progression-free survival (PFS) in patients with SCCHN treated with curative-intent non-surgical treatment who underwent baseline and response assessment FDG PET-CT and demonstrated that all four criteria had similar diagnostic performance characteristics; however, Porceddu and Deauville seemed to provide the best trade-off limiting indeterminate scores while maintaining a high negative predictive value (NPV) [106].

From the practical point of view, the role of PET-CT in determining the necessity of elective neck dissection (END) after definitive chemoradiotherapy (CCRT) was evaluated in phase 3 non-inferiority trial where 564 SCCHN patients with advanced nodal stages were randomly assigned to receive either elective neck dissection (END) within 4–8 weeks after CCRT or PET-CT scans at 12 weeks. The 2-year OS rate in PET-CT surveillance group was not inferior to the planned-surgery group (84.9 and 81.5%, respectively). PET-CT-guided surveillance also led to obviously fewer neck dissections than planned neck dissection surgery (54 and 221 cases, respectively). The PET-CT-guided surveillance would also be cost-effective [107]. Therefore, PET-CT-guided surveillance after non-surgical definitive treatment should be considered. Even though there is still a lack of the widely accepted consensus on the extent of neck surgery for residual neck disease after definitive non-surgical treatment, most of the experts suggest repeating PET-CT (preferentially), CT or MRI, or ultrasonography of the neck, 10–12 weeks after the conclusion of definitive CCRT for patients with clinical N2 and N3 diseases and consider observation if no evidence of viable residual disease exists; either observation or performing selective node dissection (SND), if post-treatment imaging studies interpret inconclusive, and performing SND or comprehensive neck dissection if residual neck disease is definitely revealed. In case of isolated neck node recurrence (without residual disease in the primary site and distant metastasis), comprehensive neck dissection is advocated, if feasible [67, 68].

4. Management of recurrent and/or metastatic HNSCC

As previously mentioned, most patients with recurrent disease are rarely suitable for salvage local therapy since such patients usually harbor extensive and intrinsically chemo- and radio-resistant diseases not amenable to salvage surgery. Furthermore, innovative radiation techniques are beneficial only in highly selective cases with very localized and low-tumor burden diseases. Among patients with metastatic disease, the prognosis is poor with a median OS of less than 1 year [108].

4.1 Cytotoxic chemotherapy

The platinum doublet therapy has been demonstrated to improve overall response rates over single-agent therapy, especially platinum in combination with either 5-fluorouracil (5-FU) or paclitaxel. Both of these combinations were shown equivalent in terms of both response rate (RR) (27% vs. 26%) and OS (8.7 vs. 8.1 months) [109]. The triplet of paclitaxel, ifosfamide, and either cisplatin or carboplatin was shown to have a much higher response rate (58 and 59%, respectively) [110, 111]. The TPF (docetaxel, cisplatin, and 5-FU) regimen was also a proven potent triplet with an RR of 44% [112]. Unfortunately, the triplets were associated with an unacceptably too high incidence of febrile neutropenia, despite the use of primary G-CSF prophylaxis.

Therefore, the triplet is not recommended in the palliative setting. Since none of these platinum-based combination regimens has been demonstrated an OS benefit over single-agent methotrexate, the platinum doublet is recommended exclusively for symptomatic and fit patients whose immediate symptomatic relief is the primary aim of management.

A substantial number of conventional single agents have been investigated. The most commonly used agents are methotrexate, cisplatin, 5-FU, and bleomyin. These agents produced a modest response rate of 15 to 30% and a very short duration of response of around 3–5 months. Pemetrexed, vinorelbine, irinotecan, a fluoropyrimidine analog (capecitabine and S-1), and a taxane (paclitaxel and docetaxel) were among the newer agents. However, the taxanes are among the most potent agents to be proven in various kinds of tumor characteristics, with RR around 20 to 43% [113].

4.2 Anti-EGFR antibodies

Overexpression of epidermal growth factor receptor (EGFR) is commonly observed in SCCHN. Since the survival benefit of cetuximab, a chimeric mouse/human monoclonal anti-EGFR antibody with concurrent RT had been investigated in locally advanced setting [114], and cetuximab was then investigated in recurrent or metastatic setting in the EXTREME trial [115]. OS was improved with the addition of cetuximab to cisplatin/5-FU (also known as the EXTREME regimen) (10.1 vs. 7.4 months; HR 0.80; $p = 0.04$). In addition, the EXTREME regimen also prolonged both PFS from 3.3 to 5.6 months and RR from 20–36% as compared with the cisplatin/5-FU combination. Another platinum doublet in combination with cetuximab, the TPEx (docetaxel, cisplatin, and cetuximab) regimen failed to demonstrate OS benefit over the EXTREME regimen in the phase 2 study, even though the overall toxicities were less than the EXTREME regimen. However, their OS was astonishingly longest among all randomized trials ever reported of 14.5 vs. 13.4 months in TPEx and EXTREME, respectively [116]. Notably, this study allowed an immune checkpoint inhibitor as a subsequent treatment upon progression. Panitumumab, a humanized monoclonal anti-EGFR antibody was also investigated in combination with cisplatin/5-FU in the SPECTRUM trial. Although panitumumab with cisplatin/5-FU led to significantly longer PFS compared with the platinum doublet alone, but it failed to show OS improvement as the primary endpoint (11.1 vs. 9 months; HR = 0.0873, $p = 0.14$) [117]. The fact that the SPECTRUM trial allowed crossover upon disease progression, while the EXTREME trial did not would be a reason for failure to demonstrate OS benefit.

4.3 Immune checkpoint inhibitors

The efficacies of various immunotherapy checkpoint inhibitors (ICI) were first assessed in the later-line setting of recurrent or metastatic SCCHN. In phase 1 KEYNOTE-012 trial, pembrolizumab resulted in a response rate of 18% and median OS of 8 months for all patients. Notably, 65% of those who responded were continuing to respond at the time of final analysis [118]. Pembrolizumab was then investigated in the phase 3 trial KEYNOTE-040 comparing with the standard of care (methotrexate, docetaxel, or cetuximab) and shown to have OS benefit among the intention-to-treat population (8.4 vs. 6.9 months; HR 0.80, $p = 0.0161$). The RR was 14.6% overall, and 17.3 and 26.6% in those with PDL-1+ (combined positive score, CPS >1%) and PDL-1+ (tumor positive score, TPS >50%), respectively. The OS was also remarkably longer among those with PDL-1+ (TPS > 50%), compared with the intent-to-treat population and those with PDL-1+ (CPS > 1%) (with a significant P-value for the interaction of 0.015) [119]. Nivolumab was assessed in the phase 3 CheckMate-141 trial [120], comparing nivolumab vs. a single-agent (methotrexate, docetaxel, or cetuximab) of an investigator's choice. As reported in the 2-year update, nivolumab improved OS significantly vs. treatment of an investigator's choice (7.7 vs. 5.1 months; HR 0.68); however, PFS was similar between treatment arms. Estimated OS rates with nivolumab were consistent regardless of the PD-L1 expression (<1% vs. ≥1%). HPV status was not the predictive marker.

Pembrolizumab was then further investigated in the first-line setting. The KEYNOTE-048 trial randomly assigned platinum-sensitive patients to receive either the EXTREME regimen, or a single-agent pembrolizumab, or a combination of the platinum (cisplatin or carboplatin)/5-fluorouracil doublet with pembrolizumab [121]. Owing to its sophisticated hierarchical data analysis using superiority or non-inferiority design according to the selected hypothesis, this trial must be interpreted cautiously. Although the PD-1 inhibitor did not provide an improvement in both PFS and RR in the overall population, monotherapy with pembrolizumab did improve OS in patients with a PD-L1+ (CPS ≥1) (12.3 vs. 10.3 months; HR 0.78, p = 0.0086). Furthermore, in the overall population, OS of single-agent pembrolizumab was determined to be non-inferior to the EXTREME regimen (11.6 vs. 10.7 months), while in patients with a PD-L1+ (CPS ≥1), pembrolizumab with platinum/chemotherapy was even superior to the EXTREME regimen (13.6 vs. 10.4 months; HR 0.77). Interestingly, the seemingly decreasing efficacy in analyses of populations with more patients having lower CPS was a concerning issue, apparently when shifting the cutoff threshold from CPS ≥20 to CPS ≥1 and then to the total populations. In the CPS <1 subgroup, there was neither OS advantage of pembrolizumab alone over EXTREME (7.9 vs. 11.3 months, HR 1.51) nor pembrolizumab/chemotherapy over EXTREME (11.3 vs. 10.7 months; HR 1.21). In the CPS 1–20 population, the benefit was confined only to the pembrolizumab/chemotherapy (12.7 vs. 9.9 months; HR 0.71) but not pembrolizumab monotherapy (10.8 vs. 10.1 months; HR 0.86). In the CPS ≥ 20 groups, pembrolizumab monotherapy yielded the longest survival, skeptically even better than pembrolizumab/chemotherapy. With debatably insufficient statistical power, the results from such *post hoc* analyses are subjected to be biased and should be speculated cautiously. The treatment-related side effects of the experimental agent were not significantly higher than EXTREME regimen. The immune-related adverse events (ir-AEs) were also as expected and manageable. Also noted, the KEYNOTE-048 excluded patients with progressive disease (PD) within six months of completion of curatively intended systemic treatment for loco-regionally advanced disease. The subgroup analysis revealed the lack of survival benefit attributable to pembrolizumab in patients presenting with local and/or regional recurrence only. Another issue of concern is the fact that the proportion of patients in the KEYNOTE-048 study who had progressive disease as the best response was indeed greater in the pembrolizumab alone group than in the EXTREME arm (41% versus 12% in the total population), irrespective of CPS explaining why PFS was not improved overall in every subgroup of CPS. Whether these results support the hyper-progression phenomenon in the pembrolizumab single-agent arm remains to be realized. This rate remains relatively consistent around 40% when anti-PD-1 agents are used alone in both the first- and second-line settings. Unexpected early disease progression seems to be unavoidable even when immunotherapy is used in combination with chemotherapy. Pembrolizumab and chemotherapy would likely act independently [122]. The provocative results from the updated data analysis on survival according to the second-line treatment from TPExtreme trial showed that the taxane-based TPEx regimen followed by an ICI in the second line provided longer OS (21.9 and 19.4 months in TPEx and EXTREME, respectively) [123]. Whether this sequential cetuximab-based and then an immune checkpoint inhibitor would be the best treatment option warrants further investigations. Those with symptomatic extensive loco-regional recurrent disease or with low PD-L1 expression would be more suitable for the platinum doublet (cisplatin/5-FU or cisplatin/docetaxel) with cetuximab as the first line. An ICI should be reserved as a second-line option in this scenario.

Other ICIs, including durvalumab, a PD-L1 inhibitor, and tremelimumab, a CTLA-4 inhibitor, has been also investigated in the second-line setting. Although the phase II HAWK trial showed promising activity of durvalumab, with a modest RR of 16.2% [124], the survival benefit of durvalumab with or without tremelimumab over chemotherapy in the overall population was not proven in the phase III EAGLE trial [125].

As revealed across the reported trials, the toxicity profile of the ICIs is significantly more favorable than conventional cytotoxic chemotherapy and is similar to what is seen with their use in other solid malignancies. They are generally well-tolerated with fatigue (20%) and nausea (9%) being the most common adverse events. Specifically, unique for these agents, the ir-AEs include thyroiditis, pneumonitis, hepatitis, colitis, nephritis, hypophysitis, myocarditis, myositis, neuritis, adrenal insufficiency, rash, and neurological toxicities. Immune-mediated thyroiditis is the most commonly seen (15%), whereas the others are less common (<5%). Most of these reactions are usually transient and minor (grades 1 and 2). Nonetheless, grade 3/4 can still occur in ~1–2% of the cases and may be fatal in some of them. Management depends on the type and severity of the ir-AEs. Thyroiditis is usually managed with thyroid hormone supplement alone, while the rests, if serious, generally involve either withholding or discontinuing treatment and administering high-dose steroids with a slow taper over weeks to months until the toxicity alleviates to grade 1 or completely resolves. Unusual cases with fatal irAEs require more potent immunosuppressive agents such as mycophenolate mofetil and infliximab (contraindicated in immune-mediated hepatitis) [126].

Despite the positive results from randomized studies showing superiority in objective response of immune checkpoint inhibitors over chemotherapy, responses are shown in 30% overall at best and half of the responders would live dramatically longer for years. On the other hand, around 40% of patients did not respond at all and some of them had unexpectedly rapid progression during treatment. Identifying the ideal biomarkers of response is therefore essential and still remains a subject under investigation. There was significant heterogeneity among the available tests for PD-L1. The definitive cutoff for PD-L1 positivity was variable across the studies and for a specific kind of tumor. Moreover, studies also differed as to whether they evaluated the PD-L1 expression on tumor cells only (tumor proportion score or TPS) or tumor cells and tumor-infiltrating immune cells (combined positive score or CPS) [127]. The tumor mutation burden (TMB), tumor immune microenvironment, HPV status [128], oral and gut microbiome [129] are among the promising alternative biomarkers that have been extensively studied; however, no definite conclusion has been proposed.

5. Conclusion

The squamous cell carcinoma of the head and neck is one of the most fatal solid malignancies. The promotion of smoking cessation, restricted alcohol consumption,

erences

ung H, Ferlay J, Siegel RL, rsanne M, Soerjomataram I, l A, et al. Global cancer statistics : GLOBOCAN estimates of lence and mortality worldwide 6 cancers in 185 countries. CA: ncer Journal for Clinicians. **71**(3):209-249

rlay J, Soerjomataram I, Dikshit R, S, Mathers C, Rebelo M, et al. Cancer ence and mortality worldwide: es, methods and major patterns in 3OCAN 2012. International Journal ncer. 2015;**136**:E359-E386

shim D, Genden E, Posner M, be M, Boffetta P. Head and neck r prevention: From primary ntion to impact of clinicians on ng burden. Annals of Oncology. **0**(5):744-756

Dermott JD, Bowles DW. niology of head and neck squamous cinomas: Impact on staging and tion strategies. Current Treatment s in Oncology. 2019;**20**(5):43

maurice C, Allen C, Barber RM, rd L, Bhutta ZA, Brenner H, et bal, regional, and national cancer ce, mortality, years of life lost, ved with disability, and disability- d life-years for 32 cancer groups, 2015: A systematic analysis for al burden of disease study. JAMA gy. 2017;**3**(4):524-548

en BT, Campbell S, Nygard M. rm incidence trends of HPV- cancers, and cases preventable by ccination: A registry-based study ay. BMJ Open. 2018;**8**:e019005

ng TZ, Hsiao JR, Tsai CR, S. Incidence trends of human papillomavirus-related head and neck cancer in Taiwan, 1995-2009. International Journal of Cancer. 2015;**137**(2):395-408

[8] Mahal BA, Catalano PJ, Haddad RI, Hanna GJ, Kass JI, Schoenfeld JD, et al. Incidence and demographic burden of HPV-associated oropharyngeal head and neck cancers in the United States. Cancer Epidemiology, Biomarkers & Prevention. 2019;**28**(10):1660-1667

[9] Gotz C, Bischof C, Wolff KD, Kolk A. Detection of HPV infection in head and neck cancers: Promise and pitfalls in the last ten years: A meta-analysis. Molecular and Clinical Oncology. 2019;**10**(1):17-28

[10] Gillison ML, Koch WM, Capone RB, Spafford M, Westra WH, Wu L, et al. Evidence for a causal association between human papillomavirus and a subset of head and neck cancers. Journal of the National Cancer Institute. 2000;**92**(9):709-720

[11] Ribeiro KB, Levi JE, Pawlita M, Koifman S, Matos E, Eluf-Neto J, et al. Low human papillomavirus prevalence in head and neck cancer: Results from two large case-control studies in high-incidence regions. International Journal of Epidemiology. 2011;**40**(2):489-502

[12] Stein AP, Saha S, Kraninger JL, Swick AD, Yu M, Lambert PF, et al. Prevalence of human papillomavirus in oropharyngeal cancer: A systematic review. Cancer Journal. 2015;**21**:138-146

[13] Kwon MJ, Kim KC, Nam ES, Cho SJ, Park HR, Min SK, et al. Programmed death ligand-1 and MET co-expression is a poor prognostic factor in gastric cancers after resection. Oncotarget. 2017;**8**(8):82399-82414

and possibly HPV vaccination would be the most economicall
control. Breakthroughs in surgical and radiotherapy techniqu
in oncological, functional, and cosmetic outcomes, especially
earlier diseases. Association with HPV is the proven prognost
although it is still not a sole predictive marker for treatment g
chemo-radiotherapy has been consistently demonstrated to b
management as the definitive treatment for patients with loc
and as the postoperative adjuvant therapy for resectable dise
features. The multi-modality treatment is very effective in ca
in exchange for significant toxicities. Flail and extreme agin
able to serious treatment-related adverse events. Carefully-t
more suitable for such patients. The recurrent or metastatic
Although the immune-checkpoint inhibitors have been able
survival outcomes, the potentially durable responses are ob
particular subgroup of patients. The researches on biomark
and proper sequence between an ICI and other proven syst
ongoing. The incorporation of novel therapies into clinical
esting area to be followed.

Funding

This article received no external funding.

Conflicts of interest

The author received honoraria from Astra-Zeneca, M
Bristol-Myers Squibb, Roche, Eisai, and Lilly for ad hoc S
participation.

Author details

Chanyoot Bandidwattanawong
Vajira Hospital, Navamindhradhiraj University, Bangk

*Address all correspondence to: chanyootmd@gmail.c

Ref

[1] S
Lav
Jem
202
inci
for 3
A Ca
2021

[2] Fe
Eser
incid
Sour
GLO
of Ca

[3] Ha
Hash
cance
preve
reduc
2019;

[4] Mc
Epider
cell ca
prever
Optior

[5] Fitz
Barreg
al. Glo
incider
years li
adjuste
1990 to
the glol
Oncolo

[6] Han
Long-te
related
HPV va
in Norw

[7] Hwa
Chang J

[14] Rieth KKS, Gill SR, Lott-Limbach AA, Merkley MA, Botero N, Allen PD, et al. Prevalence of high-risk human papillomavirus in tonsil tissue in healthy adults and colocalization in biofilm of tonsillar crypts. JAMA Otolaryngology. Head & Neck Surgery. 2018;**144**(3):231-237

[15] Mirabello L, Clarke MA, Nelson CW, Dean M, Wentzensen N, Yeager M, et al. The intersection of HPV epidemiology, genomics and mechanistic studies of HPV-mediated carcinogenesis. Viruses. 2018;**10**(2):80

[16] Herfs M, Yamamoto Y, Laury A, Wang X, Nucci MR, McLaughlin-Drubin ME, et al. A discrete population of squamocolumnar junction cells implicated in the pathogenesis of cervical cancer. Proceedings of the National Academy of Sciences of the United States of America. 2012;**109**(26):10516-10521

[17] Leemans CR, Snijders PJF, Brakenhoff RH. The molecular landscape of head and neck cancer. Nature Reviews. Cancer. 2018;**18**(5):269-282

[18] Lyford-Pike S, Peng S, Young GD, Taube JM, Westra WH, Akpeng B, et al. Evidence for a role of the PD-1:PD-L1 pathway in immune resistance of HPV-associated head and neck squamous cell carcinoma. Cancer Research. 2013;**73**(6):1733-1741

[19] Ghittoni R, Accardi R, Chiocca S, Tommasino M. Role of human papilloma viruses in carcinogenesis. Ecancermedicalscience. 2015;**9**:526

[20] Gaglia MM, Munger K. More than just oncogenes: Mechanisms of tumorigenesis by human viruses. Current Opinion in Virology. 2018;**32**:48-59

[21] Gao G, Chernock RD, Gay HA, Thorstad WL, Zhang TR, Wang H, et al. A novel RT-PCR method for quantification of human papillomavirus transcripts in archived tissues and its application in oropharyngeal cancer prognosis. International Journal of Cancer. 2013;**132**(4):882-890

[22] Lewis JS. p16 Immunohistochemistry as a standalone test for risk stratification in oropharyngeal squamous cell carcinoma. Head and Neck Pathology. 2012;**6**:S75-S82

[23] Ohta S, Uemura H, Matsui Y, Ishiguro H, Fujinami K, Kondo K, et al. Alterations of p16 and p14ARF genes and their 9p21 locus in oral squamous cell carcinoma. Oral Surgery, Oral Medicine, Oral Pathology, Oral Radiology, and Endodontics. 2009;**107**(1):81-91

[24] Kim DH, Nelson HH, Wiencke JK, Zheng S, Christiani DC, Wain JC, et al. p16(INK4a) and histology-specific methylation of CpG islands by exposure to tobacco smoke in non-small cell lung cancer. Cancer Research. 2001;**61**(8):3419-3424

[25] Saito Y, Yoshida M, Ushiku T, Omura G, Ebihara Y, Shimono T, et al. Prognostic value of p16 expression and alcohol consumption in Japanese patients with oropharyngeal squamous cell carcinoma. Cancer. 2013;**119**(11):2005-2011

[26] Huang S, Perez-Ordonez B, Liu FF, Waldron J, Ringash J, Irish J, et al. Atypical clinical behavior of p16-confirmed HPV-related oropharyngeal squamous cell carcinoma treated with radical radiotherapy. International Journal of Radiation Oncology, Biology, Physics. 2012;**82**(1):276-283

[27] Cantrell SC, Peck BW, Li G, Wei Q, Sturgis EM, Ginsberg LE. Differences in imaging characteristics of HPV-positive

and HPV negative oropharyngeal cancers: A blinded matched-pair analysis. AJNR. American Journal of Neuroradiology. 2013;**34**(10):2005-2009

[28] Trinh JM, Thomas J, Salleron J, Henrot P. Differences in clinical and imaging characteristics between p16-positive non-smokers and p16-positive smokers or p16-negative patients in oropharyngeal carcinoma. Scientific Reports. 2021;**11**(1):3314

[29] Chaturvedi AK. Epidemiology and clinical aspects of HPV in head and neck cancers. Head and Neck Pathology. 2012;**6**(Suppl 1):S16-S24

[30] Chu A, Genden E, Posner M, Sikora A. A patient centered approach to counseling patients with head and neck cancer undergoing human papillomavirus testing: A clinician's guide. The Oncologist. 2013;**18**(2):180-189

[31] Ang KK, Harris J, Wheeler R, Weber R, Rosenthal DI, Nguyen-Tân PF, et al. Human papillomavirus and survival of patients with oropharyngeal cancer. The New England Journal of Medicine. 2010;**363**:24-35

[32] Olshan AF. Epidemiology, Pathogenesis, and Prevention of Head and Neck Cancer. New York: Springer; 2010

[33] Marur S, D'Souza G, Westra WH, Forastiere A. HPV-associated head and neck cancer: A virus-related cancer epidemic. The Lancet Oncology. 2010;**11**(8):781-789

[34] Chung C, Gillison ML. Human papillomavirus in head and neck cancer: Its role in pathogenesis and clinical implications. Clinical Cancer Research. 2009;**15**(22):6758-6762

[35] Fakhry C, Westra WH, Li S, Cmelak A, Ridge JA, et al. Improved survival of pa- tients with human papillomavirus-positive head and neck squamous cell carcinoma in a prospective clinical trial. Journal of the National Cancer Institute. 2008;**100**(4):261-269

[36] Rischin D, Young RJ, Fisher R, Fox SB, Le Q-T, Peters LJ, et al. Prognostic significance of p16INK4A and human papillomavirus in patients with oropharyngeal cancer treated on TROG 02.02 phase III trial. Journal of Clinical Oncology. 2010;**28**(27):4142-4148

[37] Lassen P, Eriksen JG, Krogdahl A, Therkildsen MH, Ulhoi BP, Overgaard M, et al. The influence of HPV-associated p16 expression on accelerated fractionated radiotherapy in head and neck cancer: Evaluation of the randomised DAHANCA 6&7 trial. Radiotherapy and Oncology. 2011;**100**(1):49-55

[38] Posner M, Lorche J, Goloubeva O, Schumaker LM, Sarlis NJ, Haddad RI, et al. Survival and human papillomavirus in oropharynx cancer in TAX324: A subset analysis from an international phase III trial. Annals of Oncology. 2011;**22**(5):1071-1077

[39] Li H, Torabi SJ, Yarbrough WG, Mehra S, Osborn HA, Judson B. Association of human papillomavirus status at head and neck carcinoma subsites with overall survival. JAMA Otolaryngology. Head & Neck Surgery. 2018;**144**(6):519-525

[40] Alotaibi M, Valova V, Hänsel T, Stromberger C, Kofla G, Olze H, et al. Impact of smoking on the survival of patients with high-risk HPV-positive HNSCC: A meta-analysis. In Vivo. 2021;**35**:1017-1026

[41] Lydiatt WM, Patel SG, O'Sullivan B, Brandwein MS, Ridge JA, Migliacci JC, et al. Head and neck cancers- major changes in the American Joint Committee on Cancer Eighth Edition Cancer Staging

Manual. CA: A Cancer Journal for Clinicians. 2017;**67**(2):122-137

[42] van Gysen K, Stevens M, Guo L, Jayamanne D, Veivers D, Wignall A, et al. Validation of the 8th edition UICC/AJCC TNM staging system for HPV associated oropharyngeal cancer patients managed with contemporary chemo-radiotherapy. BMC Cancer. 2019;**19**(674):1-8

[43] Westra WH. Detection of human papillomavirus (HPV) in clinical samples: Evolving methods and strategies for the accurate determination of HPV status of head and neck carcinomas. Oral Oncology. 2014;**50**(9):771-779

[44] Nuovo GJ. In situ detection of human papillomavirus DNA after PCR-amplification. Methods in Molecular Biology. 2011;**688**:35-46

[45] Bernadt CT, Collins BT. Fine-needle aspiration biopsy of HPV-related squamous cell carcinoma of the head and neck: Current ancillary testing methods for determining HPV status. Diagnostic Cytopathology. 2017;**45**:221-229

[46] Venuti A, Paolini F. HPV detection methods in head and neck cancer. Head and Neck Pathology. 2012;**6**(Suppl 1):S63-S74

[47] Kimple RJ, Harari PM. The prognostic value of HPV in head and neck cancer patients undergoing postoperative chemoradiotherapy. Annals of Translational Medicine. 2015;**3**(Suppl1):S14

[48] El-Naggar AK, Westra WH. p16 expression as a surrogate marker for HPV-related oro- pharyngeal carcinoma: A guide for interpretative relevance and consistency. Head & Neck. 2012;**34**(4):459-461

[49] Trakoli A. IARC monographs on the evaluation of carcinogenic risks to humans. volume 99: Some aromatic amines, organic dyes, and related exposures. International Agency for Research on Cancer. Occupational Medicine. 2012;**62**(3):232

[50] Cogliano VJ, Baan R, Straif K, Grosse Y, Lauby-Secretan B, Ghissassi FE, et al. Preventable exposures associated with human cancers. Journal of the National Cancer Institute. 2011;**103**(24):1827-1839

[51] Kobayashi K, Hisamatsu K, Suzui N, Hara A, Tomita H, Miyazaki T. A review of HPV-related head and neck cancer. Journal of Clinical Medicine. 2018;**7**(9):241

[52] Mulder FJ, Pierssens DDCG, Baijens LWJ, Kremer B, Speel E-JM. Evidence for different molecular parameters in head and neck squamous cell carcinoma of nonsmokers and nondrinkers: Systematic review and meta-analysis on HPV, p16, and TP53. Head & Neck. 2020;**43**(1):303-322

[53] IARC Working Group on the Evaluation of Carcinogenic Risks to Humans. Tobacco smoke and involuntary smoking. IARC Monographs on the Evaluation of Carcinogenic Risks to Humans. 2004;**83**:1-1438

[54] Tobacco: Deadly in any form or disguise [Internet]. World Health Organization. World Health Organization; 2006 [cited 2021Dec11]. Available from: https://apps.who.int/iris/handle/10665/43465

[55] Network CGA. Comprehensive genomic characterization of head and neck squamous cell carcinomas. Nature. 2015;**517**:576-582

[56] Alexandrov LB, Nik-Zainal S, Wedge DC, Aparicio SA, Behjati S, Biankin AV, et al. Signatures of

mutational processes in human cancer. Nature. 2013;**500**:415-421

[57] Talamini R, Bosetti C, La Vecchia C, Dal Maso L, Levi F, Bidoli E, et al. Combined effect of tobacco and alcohol on laryngeal cancer risk: A case-control study. Cancer Causes & Control. 2002;**13**(10):957-964

[58] Brooks PJ, Theruvathu JA. DNA adducts from acetaldehyde: Implications for alcohol-related carcinogenesis. Alcohol. 2005;**35**:187-193

[59] León X, García J, López M, Rodriguez C, Gutierrez A, Quer M. Risk of onset of second neoplasms and successive neoplasms in patients with a head and neck index tumour. Acta Otorrinolaringologica (English Edition). 2020;**71**(1):9-15

[60] Slaughter DP, Southwick HW, Smejkal W. Field cancerization in oral stratified squamous epithelium; clinical implications of multicentric origin. Cancer. 1953;**6**:963-968

[61] Ryser MD, Lee WT, Ready NE, Leder KZ, Foo J. Quantifying the dynamics of field cancerization in tobacco-related head and neck cancer: A multiscale modeling approach. Cancer Research. 2016;**76**(24):7078-7088

[62] Giraldi L, Leoncini E, Pastorino R, Wünsch-Filho V, de Carvalho M, Lopez R, et al. Alcohol and cigarette consumption predict the mortality in patients with head and neck cancer: A pooled analysis within the International Head and Neck Epidemiology (INHANCE) Consortium. Annals of Oncology. 2017;**28**(11):2843-2851

[63] Chen AM, Chen LM, Vaughan A, Sreeraman R, Farwell DG, Luu Q, et al. Tobacco smoking during radiation therapy for head-and-neck cancer is associated with unfavorable outcome. International Journal of Radiation Oncology, Biology, Physics. 2011;**79**(2):414-419

[64] Hatcher JL, Sterba KR, Tooze JA, Day TA, Carpenter MJ, Alberg AJ, et al. Tobacco use and surgical outcomes in patients with head and neck cancer. Head & Neck. 2016;**38**(5):700-706

[65] Marin VP, Pytynia KB, Langstein HN, Dahlstrom KR, Wei Q, Sturgis EM. Serum cotinine concentration and wound complications in head and neck reconstruction. Plastic and Reconstructive Surgery. 2008;**121**(2):451-457

[66] National Comprehensive Cancer Network (NCCN Guidelines®). NCCN Clinical Practice Guidelines in Oncology. Head and Neck Cancers Version 1. 2022. 2021 Dec 8; National Comprehensive Cancer Network. [Internet]. [cited 2021Dec11]. Available from: https://www.nccn.org/professionals/physician_gls/pdf/head-and-neck.pdf

[67] Keam B, Machiels JP, Kim HR, Licitra L, Golusinski W, Gregoire V, et al. Pan-Asian adaptation of the EHNS–ESMO–ESTRO clinical practice guidelines for the diagnosis, treatment and follow-up of patients with squamous cell carcinoma of the head and neck. ESMO Open. 2021;**6**(6):100309

[68] Forastiere AA, Weber RS, Trotti A. Organ preservation for advanced larynx cancer: Issues and outcomes. Journal of Clinical Oncology. 2015;**33**:3262-3268

[69] Patel SA, Qureshi MM, Dyer MA, Jalisi S, Grillone G, Truong MT. Comparing surgical and nonsurgical larynx-preserving treatments with total laryngectomy for locally advanced laryngeal cancer. Cancer. 2019;**125**(19):3367-3377

[70] Paleri V, Urbano TG, Mehanna RC, Lancaster J, Roques T, et al. Management of neck metastases in head and neck cancer: United Kingdom National Multidisciplinary Guidelines. The Journal of Laryngology and Otology. 2016;**130**(Suppl. S2):S161-S169

[71] White H, Ford S, Bush B, Holsinger FC, Moore E, Ghanem T, et al. Salvage surgery for recurrent cancers of the oropharynx: Comparing TORS with standard open surgical approaches. JAMA Otolaryngology. Head & Neck Surgery. 2013;**139**(8):773-778

[72] De Almeida JR, Li R, Magnuson JS, Smith RV, Moore E, Lawson G, et al. Oncologic outcomes after transoral robotic surgery: A multi-institutional study. JAMA Otolaryngology. Head & Neck Surgery. 2015;**141**(12):1043-1051

[73] Braakhuis BJ, Brakenhoff RH, Leemans CR. Treatment choice for locally advanced head and neck cancers on the basis of risk factors: Biological risk factors. Annals of Oncology. 2012;**23**(Suppl 10):x173-x177

[74] Cooper JS, Pajak TF, Forastiere A, Jacobs J, Fu KK, Ang KK, et al. Precisely defining high-risk operable head and neck tumors based on RTOG #85-03 and #88-24: Targets for postoperative radiochemotherapy? Head & Neck. 1998;**20**(7):588-594

[75] Hosni A, Huang SH, Chiu K, Xu W, Su J, Bayley A, et al. Predictors of early recurrence prior to planned postoperative radiation therapy for oral cavity squamous cell carcinoma and outcomes following salvage intensified radiation therapy. International Journal of Radiation Oncology, Biology, Physics. 2019;**103**(2):363-373

[76] Ang KK, Trotti A, Brown BW, Garden AS, Foote RL, Morrison WH, et al. Randomized trial addressing risk features and time factors of surgery plus radiotherapy in advanced head-and-neck cancer. International Journal of Radiation Oncology, Biology, Physics. 2001;**51**(3):571-578

[77] Noble AR, Greskovich JF, Han J, Reddy CA, Nwizu TI, Khan MF, et al. Risk factors associated with disease recurrence in patients with stage III/IV squamous cell carcinoma of the oral cavity treated with surgery and postoperative radiotherapy. Anticancer Research. 2016;**36**(2):785-792

[78] International Consortium for Outcome Research (ICOR) in Head and Neck Cancer, Ebrahimi A, Gil Z, Amit M, Yen TC, Liao CT, et al. Primary tumor staging for oral cancer and a proposed modification incorporating depth of invasion: An international multicenter retrospective study. JAMA Otolaryngology. Head & Neck Surgery. 2014;**140**(12):1138-1148

[79] Bernier J, Domenge C, Ozsahin M, Matuszewska K, Lefèbvre JL, Greiner RH, et al. European Organization for Research and Treatment of Cancer Trial 22931. Postoperative irradiation with or without concomitant chemotherapy for locally advanced head and neck cancer. The New England Journal of Medicine. 2004;**350**(19):1945-1952

[80] Cooper JS, Pajak TF, Forastiere AA, Jacobs J, Campbell BH, Saxman SB, et al. Radiation Therapy Oncology Group 9501/Intergroup. Postoperative concurrent radiotherapy and chemotherapy for high-risk squamous-cell carcinoma of the head and neck. The New England Journal of Medicine. 2004;**350**(19):1937-1944

[81] Bernier J, Cooper JS, Pajak TF, van Glabbeke M, Bourhis J, Forastiere A, et al.

Defining risk levels in locally advanced head and neck cancers: A comparative analysis of concurrent postoperative radiation plus chemotherapy trials of the EORTC (#22931) and RTOG (# 9501). Head & Neck. 2005;**27**(10):843-850

[82] Bachaud JM, Cohen-Jonathan E, Alzieu C, David JM, Serrano E, Daly-Schveitzer N. Combined postoperative radio- therapy and weekly cisplatin infusion for locally advanced head and neck carcinoma: Final report of a randomized trial. International Journal of Radiation Oncology, Biology, Physics. 1996;**36**(5):999-1004

[83] Kiyota N, Tahara M, Fujii H, Yamazaki T, Mitani H, Iwae S, et al. Phase II/III trial of post-operative chemoradiotherapy comparing 3-weekly cisplatin with weekly cisplatin in high-risk patients with squamous cell carcinoma of head and neck (JCOG1008). Journal of Clinical Oncology. 2020;**38**(15 Suppl):Abstract 6502

[84] Margalit DN, Sacco AG, Cooper JS, Ridge JA, Bakst RL, Beadle BM, et al. Systematic review of postoperative therapy for resected squamous cell carcinoma of the head and neck: Executive summary of the American Radium Society appropriate use criteria. Head & Neck. 2021;**43**(1):367-391

[85] Matuschek C, Haussmann J, Bölke E, Gripp S, Schuler PJ, Tamaskovics B, et al. Accelerated vs. conventionally fractionated adjuvant radiotherapy in high-risk head and neck cancer: A meta-analysis. Radiation Oncology. 2018;**13**(1):195

[86] Sanguineti G, Richetti A, Bignardi M, Corvo' R, Gabriele P, Sormani MP, et al. Accelerated versus conventional fractionated postoperative radiotherapy for advanced head and neck cancer: Results of a multicenter Phase III study. International Journal of Radiation Oncology, Biology, Physics. 2005;**61**(3):762-771

[87] Lacas B, Carmel A, Landais C, Wong SJ, Licitra L, Tobias JS, et al. Meta-analysis of chemotherapy in head and neck cancer (MACH-NC): An update on 107 randomized trials and 19,805 patients, on behalf of MACH-NC Group. Radiotherapy and Oncology. 2021;**156**:281-293

[88] Gau M, Karabajakian A, Reverdy T, Neidhardt E-M, Fayette J. Induction chemotherapy in head and neck cancers: Results and controversies. Oral Oncology. 2019;**95**:164-169

[89] Petit C, Lacas B, Pignon J-P, Le QT, Grégoire V, Grau C, et al. Chemotherapy and radiotherapy in locally advanced head and neck cancer: An individual patient data network meta-analysis. The Lancet Oncology. 2021;**22**(5):727-736

[90] Adelstein DJ, Ismaila N, Ku JA, Burtness B, Swiecicki PL, Mell L, et al. Role of treatment deintensification in the management of p16+ oropharyngeal cancer: ASCO provisional clinical opinion. Journal of Clinical Oncology. 2019;**37**(18):1578-1589

[91] Nichols AC, Lang P, Prisman E, Berthelet E, Tran E, Hamilton S, et al. Treatment de-escalation for HPV-associated oropharyngeal squamous cell carcinoma with radiotherapy vs. trans-oral surgery (ORATOR2): Study protocol for a randomized phase II trial. BMC Cancer. 2020;**20**(1):125

[92] Ferris RL, Flamand Y, Weinstein GS, Li S, Quon H, Mehra R, et al. Phase II randomized trial of transoral surgery and low-dose intensity modulated radiation therapy in resectable p16+ locally advanced oropharynx cancer: An ECOG-ACRIN cancer research group trial

(E3311). Journal of Clinical Oncology. 2021;**26**:JCO2101752

[93] Owadally W, Hurt C, Timmins H, Parsons E, Townsend S, Patterson J, et al. PATHOS: A phase II/III trial of risk-stratified, reduced intensity adjuvant treatment in patients undergoing transoral surgery for Human papillomavirus (HPV) positive oropharyngeal cancer. BMC Cancer. 2015;**15**:602

[94] Yom SS, Torres-Saavedra P, Caudell JJ, Waldron JN, Gillison ML, Xia P, et al. Reduced-dose radiation therapy for HPV-associated oropharyngeal carcinoma (NRG Oncology HN002). Journal of Clinical Oncology. 2021;**39**(9):956-965

[95] Gillison ML, Trotti AM, Harris J, Eisbruch A, Harari PM, Adelstein DJ, et al. Radiotherapy plus cetuximab or cisplatin in human papillomavirus-positive oropharyngeal cancer (NRG Oncology RTOG 1016): A randomised, multicentre, non-inferiority trial. Lancet. 2019;**393**(10166):40-50

[96] Mehanna H, Robinson M, Hartley A, Kong A, Foran B, Fulton-Lieuw T, et al. De-ESCALaTE HPV Trial Group. Radiotherapy plus cisplatin or cetuximab in low-risk human papillomavirus-positive oropharyngeal cancer (De-ESCALaTE HPV): An open-label randomised controlled phase 3 trial. Lancet. 2019;**393**(10166):51-60

[97] Rischin D, King M, Kenny L, Porceddu S, Wratten C, Macann A, et al. Randomized trial of radiation therapy with weekly cisplatin or cetuximab in low-risk HPV-associated oropharyngeal cancer (TROG 12.01) - A trans-tasman radiation oncology group study. International Journal of Radiation Oncology, Biology, Physics. 2021;**111**(4):876-886

[98] Denaro N, Merlano MC, Russi EG. Follow-up in head and neck cancer: Do more does it mean do better? A systematic review and our proposal based on our experience. Clinical and Experimental Otorhinolaryngology. 2016;**9**(4):287-297

[99] Lowe VJ, Duan F, Subramaniam RM, Sicks JD, Romanoff J, Bartel T, et al. Multicenter trial of [^{18}F] fluorodeoxyglucose positron emission tomography/computed tomography staging of head and neck cancer and negative predictive value and surgical impact in the N0 neck: Results from ACRIN 6685. Journal of Clinical Oncology. 2019;**37**(20):1704-1712

[100] Mehanna H, McConkey CC, Rahman JK, Wong WL, Smith AF, Nutting C, et al. PET-NECK: A multicentre randomised Phase III non-inferiority trial comparing a positron emission tomography-computerised tomography-guided watch-and-wait policy with planned neck dissection in the management of locally advanced (N2/N3) nodal metastases in patients with squamous cell head and neck cancer. Health Technology Assessment. 2017;**21**(17):1-122

[101] Kale H, Rath TJ. Chapter 3 The role of PET/CT in squamous cell carcinoma of the head and neck. Seminars in Ultrasound, CT, and MR. 2017;**38**(5):479-494

[102] Sjövall J, Bitzén U, Kjellén E, Nilsson P, Wahlberg P, Brun E. Qualitative interpretation of PET scans using a Likert scale to assess neck node response to radiotherapy in head and neck cancer. European Journal of Nuclear Medicine and Molecular Imaging. 2016;**43**(4):609-616

[103] Koksel Y, Gencturk M, Spano A, Reynolds M, Roshan S, Caycı Z. Utility

of Likert scale (Deauville criteria) in assessment of Chemoradiotherapy response of primary oropharyngeal squamous cell Cancer site. Clinical Imaging. 2019;**55**:89-94

[104] Huang YC, Li SH, Lu HI, Hsu CC, Wang YM, Lin WC, et al. Post-chemoradiotherapy FDG PET with qualitative interpretation criteria for outcome stratification in esophageal squamous cell carcinoma. PLoS One. 2019;**14**(1):e0210055

[105] Zhong J, Sundersingh M, Dyker K, Currie S, Vaidyanathan S, Prestwich R, et al. Post-treatment FDG PET-CT in head and neck carcinoma: Comparative analysis of 4 qualitative interpretative criteria in a large patient cohort. Scientific Reports. 2020;**10**:4086

[106] Mehanna H, Wong WL, McConkey CC, Rahman JK, Robinson M, Hartley AG, et al. PET-NECK trial management group. PET-CT surveillance versus neck dissection in advanced head and neck cancer. The New England Journal of Medicine. 2016;**374**(15):1444-1454

[107] Price KA, Cohen EE. Current treatment options for metastatic head and neck cancer. Current Treatment Options in Oncology. 2012;**13**(1):35-46

[108] Gibson MK, Li Y, Murphy B, Hussain MHA, DeConti RC, Ensley J, et al. Randomized phase III evaluation of cisplatin plus fluorouracil versus cisplatin plus paclitaxel in advanced head and neck cancer (E1395): An intergroup trial of the eastern cooperative oncology group. Journal of Clinical Oncology. 2005;**23**(15):3562-3567

[109] Shin DM, Glisson BS, Khuri FR, Ginsberg L, Papadimitrakopoulou V, Lee JJ, et al. Phase II trial of paclitaxel, ifosfamide, and cisplatin in patients with recurrent head and neck squamous cell carcinoma. Journal of Clinical Oncology. 1998;**16**(4):1325-1330

[110] Shin DM, Khuri FR, Glisson BS, Ginsberg L, Papadimitrakopoulou VM, Clayman G, et al. Phase II study of paclitaxel, ifosfamide, and carboplatin in patients with recurrent or metastatic head and neck squamous cell carcinoma. Cancer. 2001;**91**(7):1316-1323

[111] Janinis J, Papadakou M, Xidakis E, Boukis H, Poulis A, Panagos G, et al. Combination chemotherapy with docetaxel, cisplatin, and 5-fluorouracil in previously treated patients with advanced/recurrent head and neck cancer: A phase II feasibility study. American Journal of Clinical Oncology. 2000;**23**(2):128-131

[112] Molin Y, Fayette J. Current chemotherapies for recurrent/metastatic head and neck cancer. Anti-Cancer Drugs. 2011;**22**(7):621-625

[113] Bonner JA, Harari PM, Giralt J, Azarnia N, Shin DM, Cohen RB, et al. Radiotherapy plus cetuximab for squamous-cell carcinoma of the head and neck. The New England Journal of Medicine. 2006;**354**(6):567-578

[114] Vermorken JB, Mesia R, Rivera F, Remenar E, Kawecki A, Rottey S, et al. Platinum-based chemotherapy plus cetuximab in head and neck cancer. The New England Journal of Medicine. 2008;**359**(11):1116-1127

[115] Guigay J, Auperin A, Fayette J, Saada-Bouzid E, Lafond C, Taberna M, et al. Cetuximab, docetaxel, and cisplatin versus platinum, fluorouracil, and cetuximab as first-line treatment in patients with recurrent or metastatic head and neck squamous-cell carcinoma (GORTEC 2014-01 TPExtreme):

A multicentre, open-label, randomised, phase 2 trial. The Lancet Oncology. 2021;**22**(4):463-475

[116] Vermorken JB, Stohlmacher-Williams J, Davidenko I, Licitra L, Winquist E, Villanueva C, et al. Cisplatin and fluorouracil with or without panitumumab in patients with recurrent or metastatic squamous-cell carcinoma of the head and neck (SPECTRUM): An open-label phase 3 randomised trial. The Lancet Oncology. 2013;**14**(8):697-710

[117] Seiwert TY, Burtness B, Mehra R, Weiss J, Berger R, Eder JP, et al. Safety and clinical activity of pembrolizumab for treatment of recurrent or metastatic squamous cell carcinoma of the head and neck (KEYNOTE-012): An open-label, multicentre, phase 1b trial. The Lancet Oncology. 2016;**17**(7):956-965

[118] Cohen EEW, Soulieres D, Le Tourneau C, Dinis J, Licitra L, Ahn M-J, et al. Pembrolizumab versus methotrexate, docetaxel, or cetuximab for recurrent or metastatic head-and-neck squamous cell carcinoma (KEYNOTE-040): A randomised, open-label, phase 3 study. Lancet. 2018;**393**(10167):156-167

[119] Ferris RL, Blumenschein G, Fayette J, Guigay J, Colevas AD, Licitra L, et al. Two-year update from CheckMate 141: Outcomes with nivolumab (Nivo) vs investigator's choice (IC) in recurrent or metastatic (R/M) squamous cell carcinoma of the head and neck (SCCHN) in the overall population and PD-L1 subgroups. International Journal of Radiation Oncology, Biology, Physics. 2018;**100**(5):LBA10

[120] Burtness B, Harrington KJ, Greil R, Soulières D, Tahara M, de Castro G Jr, et al. Pembrolizumab alone or with chemotherapy versus cetuximab with chemotherapy for recurrent or metastatic squamous cell carcinoma of the head and neck (KEYNOTE-048): A randomised, open-label, phase 3 study. Lancet. 2019;**394**(10212):1915-1928

[121] Szturz P, Vermorken JB. Translating KEYNOTE-048 into practice recommendations for head and neck cancer. Annals of Translational Medicine. 2020;**8**(15):975

[122] Guigay J, Auperin A, Fayette J, Saada-Bouzid E, Lafond C, Taberna M, et al. TPExtreme randomized trial: Quality of Life (QoL) and survival according to second-line treatments in patients with recurrent/metastatic head and neck squamous cell carcinoma (R/M HNSCC). Journal of Clinical Oncology. 2020;**38**(15 Suppl):Abstract 6507

[123] Zandberg DP, Algazi AP, Jimeno A, Good JS, Fayette J, Bouganim N, et al. Durvalumab for recurrent or metastatic head and neck squamous cell carcinoma: Results from a single-arm, phase II study in patients with ≥25% tumour cell PD-L1 expression who have progressed on platinum-based chemotherapy. European Journal of Cancer. 2019;**107**:142-152

[124] Ferris RL, Haddad R, Even C, Tahara M, Dvorkin M, Ciuleanu TE, et al. Durvalumab with or without tremelimumab in patients with recurrent or metastatic head and neck squamous cell carcinoma: EAGLE, a randomized, open-label phase III study. Annals of Oncology. 2020;**31**(7):942-950

[125] Schneider BJ, Naidoo J, Santomasso BD, Lacchetti C, Adkins S, Anadkat M, et al. Management of immune-related adverse events in patients treated with immune checkpoint inhibitor therapy: American Society of Clinical Oncology Clinical Practice Guideline Update. Journal of Clinical Oncolology. 2021;**39**:4073-4126

[126] Udall M, Rizzo M, Kenny J, Doherty J, Dahm SA, Robbins P, et al. PD-L1 diagnostic tests: A systematic literature review of scoring algorithms and test-validation metrics. Diagnostic Pathology. 2018;**13**(12):1-12

[127] Canning M, Guo G, Yu M, Myint C, Groves MW, Byrd JK, et al. Heterogeneity of the head and neck squamous cell carcinoma immune landscape and its impact on immunotherapy. Frontiers in Cell and Development Biology. 2019;**7**:52

[128] Gopalakrishnan V, Spencer CN, Nezi L, Reuben A, Andrews MC, Karpinets TV, et al. Gut microbiome modulates response to anti-PD-1 immunotherapy in melanoma patients. Science. 2018;**359**:97-103

[129] Bandidwattanawong C, Chalongphobsinchai S, Tantiwattana T. Squamous cell carcinoma of head and neck in vajira hospital: The outcomes in a real-world practice. Journal of Medical Association of Thailand. 2020;**103**(7):702-710

Chapter 7

Squamous Cell Carcinoma of the Eyelid and Ocular Surface

Jin-Jhe Wang, Yueh-Ju Tsai and Chau-Yin Chen

Abstract

Squamous cell carcinoma that arises from the eye and its adnexa has gained more attention as the incidence rises globally. The malignancy has a broad spectrum of clinical manifestations and, if not properly treated, may affect both vision and life. In this chapter, we will go over the squamous cell carcinoma that occurs on the ocular surface and its adnexa, including the eyelid and lacrimal apparatus. We would like to introduce the epidemiology, pathophysiology, diagnosis methods, recurrence and prognosis of this squamous neoplasm. Furthermore, we review most of the current treatment strategies for squamous cell carcinoma of the eyelid and ocular surface ranging from medical to surgical measures.

Keywords: eyelid squamous cell carcinoma, ocular surface squamous neoplasm, squamous cell carcinoma of lacrimal apparatus

1. Introduction

Squamous cell carcinoma (SCC) of the eye is an invasive epithelial malignancy and involves the periocular skin, ocular surface and lacrimal apparatus [1]. Over the past four decades, there has been a progressive rise in the global incidence of SCC on account of increased exposure to carcinogens such as ultraviolet (UV) radiation, cigarette smoking, immunosuppressive drugs or human papillomavirus (HPV) infection [1–3]. The tumor comprises a large and diverse spectrum of conditions and threatens both vision and life. Diagnosis and management of patients with such malignant ophthalmic tumors present additional challenges.

2. Epidemiology

Eyelid SCC is the second most common periocular skin malignancy, far exceeded by basal cell carcinoma (BCC) which is 10–13 times more common [4, 5]. The reported incidence of SCC of the eyelid is 0.09 to 2.42 cases per 100,000 persons per year, representing 3.4–12.6% of all types of malignant eyelid neoplasms [6]. A longitudinal study in England has shown that the age-standardized incidence of SCC has increased approximately 2% per year between 2000 and 2014 [3]. It mainly presents in the seventh decade of life with a male predominance (1.83:1) [7].

Ocular surface SCC is the most common primary ocular neoplasm with reported incidence from 0.3 to 1.9 per 100,000 persons per year, accounting 4–29% of all oculo-orbital tumors [8–10].

Primary lacrimal sac/duct malignancies are very rare with SCC being the most frequently reported neoplasm [11]. In one study, only 38 out of 3865 (0.98%) specimens of lacrimal sac biopsy showed malignant [12].

3. Demographics and risk factors

SCC is prevalent in the elderly and more frequent among men than women [1, 3]. Typically, SCC affects individuals with a fair complexion and a history of chronic sunlight exposure, which is reflected in an increased risk in white populations [3]. Advanced age and cumulative UV radiation are the major risk factors for SCC formation [6, 13, 14]. There is a doubling in the incidence of SCC with each 10-degree reduction in latitude and every decade increase over the age of sixty [3, 15]. Ionizing radiation, exposure to chemicals (arsenic, polycyclic hydrocarbons and psoralen), high fat diet, cigarette smoking, and infection of HPV also contribute to the formation of SCC [5]. Higher rate of SCC development has been observed in those with immunosuppression secondary to organ transplantation and acquired immunodeficiency syndrome (AIDS) [16, 17]. Studies have shown that the risk of developing SCC varies with the types of transplants and the time intervals following transplantation [17–19]. Other intrinsic factors predisposing to SCC include preexisting skin neoplasms, chronic cutaneous inflammatory lesions (such as nonhealing wounds, ulcers, burns, scars and sinus tracts), and genetic skin disorders (such as xeroderma pigmentosum, epidermodysplasia verruciformis and albinism) [1, 7, 20].

4. Pathogenesis and pathology

SCC may arise de novo or from preexisting actinic keratosis or carcinoma in situ (Bowen disease) [1, 7, 21]. Conjunctival intraepithelial neoplasia (CIN) refers to varying degrees of conjunctival epithelial dysplasia. CIN that involves the entire epithelium is referred to as carcinoma in situ. In some cases of squamous cell papilloma, they have been found to grow quite large, covering the surface of the cornea and simulating a squamous cell carcinoma. Most cases of squamous cell papilloma are benign tumor, but its potential for malignant transformation has yet to be studied (**Figures 1** and **2**). Development of such malignancy undergoes a multi-step process of carcinogenesis involving mutations of genes (such as TP53, CDKN2A, NOTCH1 and NOTCH2, EGFR and TERT) and molecular pathways (RAS–RAF–MEK–ERK and PI3K-AKT–mTOR), epigenetic modifications, viral oncogenesis, and microenvironmental changes [18, 22]. Inactivation of the p53 tumor suppressor gene results in altered apoptosis and clonal proliferation of keratinocytes [1, 18]. Moreover, upregulation of matrix metalloproteinases (MMPs) and other factors account for the invasive activity associated with tumor progression [22].

Histologically, SCC is characterized by full-thickness atypia of squamous cells with increased mitotic activity, pleomorphism, and prominent nuclei. The tumor is classified as carcinoma in situ when it is confined to the basement membrane, and as invasive SCC when it extends deep to the dermis or stroma. In a well-differentiated tumor, the cells form nests and strands and exhibit polygonal with abundant eosinophilic

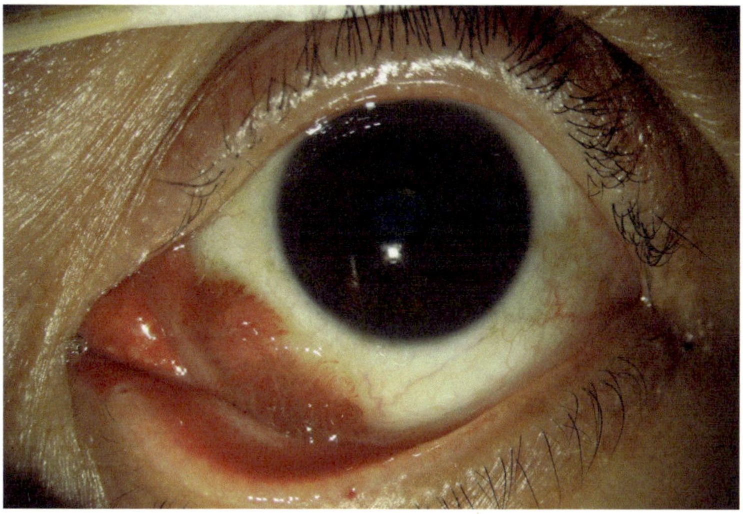

Figure 1.
Periocular squamous cell papilloma with focal mild dysplasia.

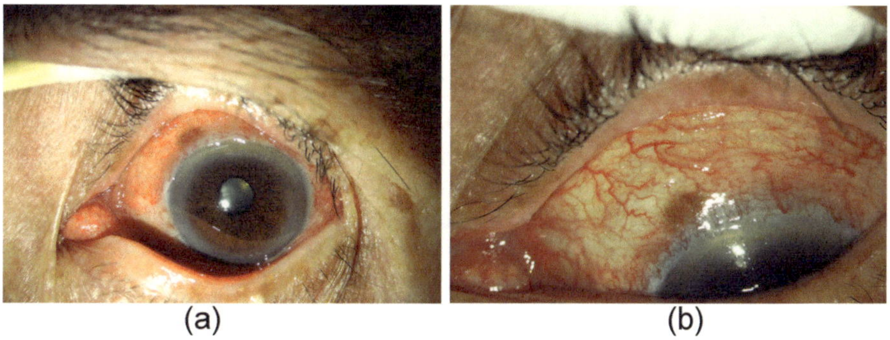

Figure 2.
Diffused type of conjunctival squamous cell carcinoma (conjunctival intraepithelial neoplasm). a, gross view. b, high magnification (X2 original).

cytoplasm and hyperchromatic nuclei. Dyskeratosis, keratin pearls, intercellular bridges are more prominent. Poorly differentiated SCC presents high pleomorphism with anaplastic cells, little keratinization and loss of intercellular bridges. Other variants include spindle and adenoid SCC [1]. Immunohistochemical studies may be useful in diagnosis as cells are positive for epithelial membrane antigen (EMA), cytokeratin, prekeratin, AE1/AE3, MNF16, p63 [5, 23, 24]. Stains for CAM5.2, Ber-EP4, adipophilin, lysozyme, S100 protein and desmin are negative [5, 24, 25].

5. Clinical presentation

5.1 Cutaneous SCC of the eyelid and periocular skin

The appearance of cutaneous SCC (cSCC) has a broad spectrum and may be indistinguishable from various benign and malignant lesions. Collision tumor,

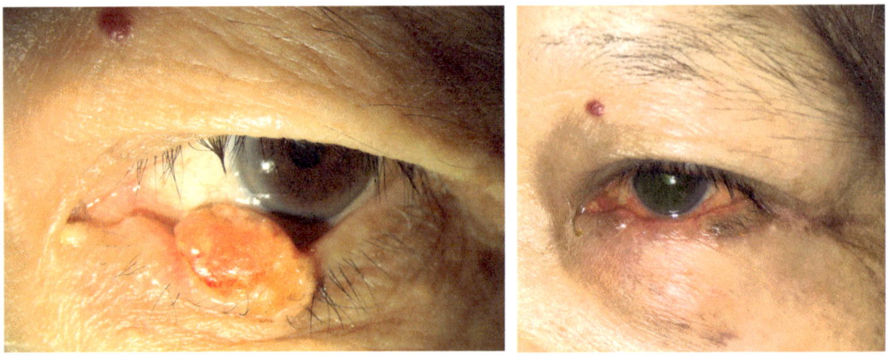

(a) (b)

Figure 3.
Collision tumor of squamous cell carcinoma and sebaceous cell carcinoma coincident in a single mass. a, preoperative photograph. b, postoperative status with reconstruction.

a neoplastic lesion comprised of two or more distinct cell populations that maintain distinct borders, which is rare but well documented in the eyelid (**Figure 3**) [23]. Studies had reported that the accuracy of preoperative clinical diagnosis of cSCC is 51–62.7% [6, 7, 26]. The tumor has a predilection for the lower eyelid and medial can thus, similar to basal cell carcinomas (BCCs). However, cSCC is more likely to involve the upper eyelid than is BCC (**Figure 4**). SCC of the eyelids grows more rapidly and aggressively than does BCC. The tumor typically appears as a slightly raised nodule or plaque with irregular margins and overlying scaling, crusting, induration, keratinization, or ulceration. Some may feature cutaneous horn, papillomatous lesion, and large fungating growth. The periocular architecture may be distorted and madarotic. The surface vascularization or telangiectasia is usually absent.

Eyelid SCC has potential for local extension with tissue destruction and perineural infiltration which may facilitate intraorbital and intracranial spread with associated cranial neuropathies. This occurs in 4–8% of cases [7, 27]. Unlike BCC, SCC tends to metastasize to regional lymph nodes and distant sites through lymphatic and haematogenous routes. The rate of metastasis ranges from 1–24% depending on tumor size, length of follow up and underlying risk factors [28, 29].

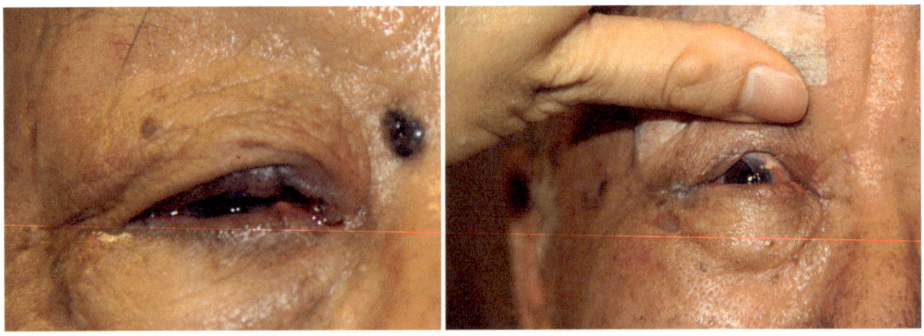

(a) (b)

Figure 4.
Cutaneous SCC of the eyelid. a, preoperative photograph. b, postoperative status with reconstruction.

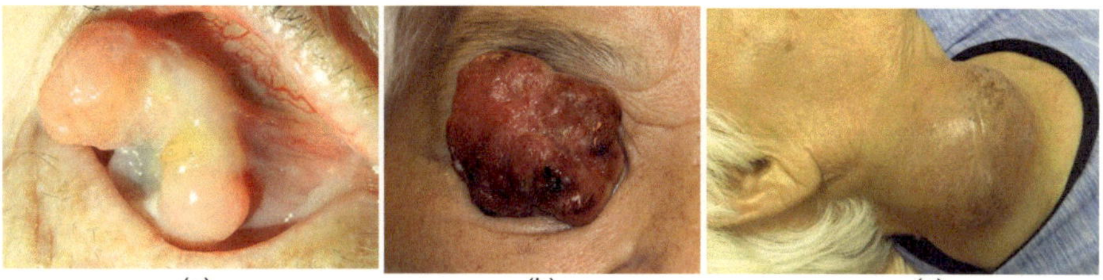

(a) (b) (c)

Figure 5.
Advanced spindle squamous cell carcinoma. A, primary site. B, after one year without treatment. C, submandibular lymph node metastasis.

5.2 SCC of conjunctiva and cornea

Conjunctival or corneal SCC belongs to the disease spectrum of ocular surface squamous neoplasia (OSSN). It appears as a fleshy, elevated plaque-like lesion usually at the limbus and bulbar conjunctiva within the interpalpebral fissure zone [30]. There are three common morphologic patterns: leukoplakic, papillomatous and gelatinous [31]. Superficial feeder vasculature and pigmentation of the lesion may be prominent, but some tumors may appear avascular. The tumor may cause ocular irritation, foreign body sensation, pruritus, conjunctival congestion, decreased vision and even diplopia.

Although, the metastatic disease is rare, local invasion through corneoscleral lamella into the anterior chamber occurs in about 40% of cases [32, 33]. Mucoepidermoid carcinoma and spindle cell carcinoma (**Figure 5**) are other rare variants of conjunctival SCC which tend to be more aggressive and more likely to invade the globe or orbit [30, 34]. The incidence of intraocular spread by conjunctival SCC is reported up to 13% and orbital invasion about 12–16% [35–37].

5.3 SCC of lacrimal drainage system

The clinical manifestations of lacrimal sac tumors are featureless such as chronic epiphora and recurrent dacryocystitis. However, a firm, nonreducible, nontender mass with insidious growth above the medial canthal tendon should prompt the suspicion of possible malignancy [38, 39]. The tumor may invade the skin and produce ulceration and spontaneous bleeding.

Metastasis to regional lymph nodes may also occur. When regional or distant metastases are present in all types of ophthalmic SCC, the prognosis is poor, and the mortality is high [1].

6. Tumor staging

To achieve minimizing the rate of recurrence, a complete pre-op assessment must be made, including a highly precise clinical approach to the diagnostic: whether the lesion is circumscribed or diffuse, bilateral or unilateral, suspected to be pre-cancerous or malign. The extension of the tumor must also be assessed, determining the existence of intra-ocular and/or intra-orbital invasion, carrying out palpation of regional lymphatics and, when considered appropriate, a systemic extension study for detecting metastasis.

Category	Definition
Primary tumor (T)	
TX	Primary tumor cannot be assessed
T0	No evidence of primary tumor
Tis	Carcinoma in situ
T1	Tumor ≤10 mm in greatest dimension
T1a	Tumor does not invade the tarsal plate or eyelid margin
T1b	Tumor invades the tarsal plate or eyelid margin
T1c	Tumor involves full thickness of the eyelid
T2	Tumor >10 mm but ≤20 mm in greatest dimension
T2a	Tumor does not invade the tarsal plate or eyelid margin
T2b	Tumor invades the tarsal plate or eyelid margin
T2c	Tumor involves full thickness of the eyelid
T3	Tumor >20 mm but ≤30 mm in greatest dimension
T3a	Tumor does not invade the tarsal plate or eyelid margin
T3b	Tumor invades the tarsal plate or eyelid margin
T3c	Tumor involves full thickness of the eyelid
T4	Any eyelid tumor that invades adjacent ocular, orbital, or facial structures
T4a	Tumor invades ocular or intraorbital structures
T4b	Tumor invades (or erodes through) the bony walls of the orbit or extends to the paranasal sinuses or invades the lacrimal sac / nasolacrimal duct or brain
Regional lymph nodes (N)	
NX	Regional lymph nodes cannot be assessed
N0	No evidence of lymph node involvement
N1	Metastasis in a single ipsilateral regional lymph node, ≤ 3 cm in greatest dimension
N1a	Metastasis in a single ipsilateral regional lymph node based on clinical evaluation or imaging findings
N1b	Metastasis in a single ipsilateral regional lymph node based on lymph node biopsy
N2	Metastasis in a single ipsilateral regional lymph node, > 3 cm in greatest dimension, or in bilateral or contralateral lymph nodes
N2a	Metastasis documented based on clinical evaluation or imaging findings
N2b	Metastasis documented based on microscopic findings on lymph node biopsy
Distant metastasis (M)	
M0	No distant metastasis
M1	Distant metastasis

AJCC, American Joint Committee on Cancer.

Table 1.
Staging for eyelid carcinoma according to AJCC 8th edition.

Category	Definition
Primary tumor (T)	
TX	Primary tumor cannot be assessed
T0	No evidence of primary tumor
Tis	Carcinoma in situ
T1	Tumor ≤5 mm. Or less in greatest dimension
T2	Tumor >5 mm. In greatest dimension, without invasion of adjacent structures
T3	Tumor invades adjacent structures (excluding the orbit)
T4	Tumor invades the orbit with or without further extension
T4a	Tumor invades the orbital soft tissues, without bone invasion
T4b	Tumor invades bone
T4c	Tumor invades adjacent paranasal sinuses
T4d	Tumor invades brain
Regional lymph nodes (N)	
NX	Regional lymph nodes cannot be assessed
N0	No regional lymph node metastasis
N1	Regional lymph node metastasis
Distant metastasis (M)	
M0	No distant metastasis
M1	Distant metastasis
AJCC, American Joint Committee on Cancer.	

Table 2.
Staging for conjunctival carcinoma according to AJCC 7th edition.

Clinical staging is based on the assessment of cancer by inspection; slit-lamp examination, palpation of regional nodes, and clinical photography are used, as well as preoperative ultrasound biomicroscopy (UBM) and (Optical Coherence Tomograph) OCT when the intraocular invasion is suspected. Radiological examination (CT, magnetic resonance imaging [MRI], and PET/CT) can be used to examine regional node status, paranasal sinuses, orbit, brain, and chest. Ongoing studies are designed to clarify the role of sentinel node biopsy in the accurate staging of invasive squamous cell carcinoma [40].

TNM staging also includes clinical classification and pathological classification as outlined by the American Joint Committee on Cancer (AJCC), this staging applies to squamous carcinomas with the natural history of lymphatic spread to regional nodes, the possibility of hematogenous metastases, as well as subsequent locoregional disease and metastatic disease. **Tables 1** and **2** are the staging of eyelid SCC and ocular surface SCC, respectively.

7. Management

7.1 Surgical treatment

7.1.1 Conjunctival SCC treatment

The management of CIN or SCC in the ocular surface varies with the extent or recurrence of the lesion. To completely destroy or extirpate the tumor through surgery and adjuvating treatments (cryotherapy, topical chemotherapy, radiotherapy) remains the widely accepted treatment strategy for primary lesion after precise histopathological confirmation.

Most of the primary conjunctival squamous cell carcinoma arises in the interpalpebral area near the limbus and the surgical technique for limbal tumors is different than that for forniceal tumors [41–44].

In general, for tumors that are circumscribed, limbar or conjunctival bulbar, complete extirpation (excisional biopsy) with the smallest possible amount of manipulation and a resection margin of 3–5 mm could be sufficient treatment. Limbal neoplasms possibly can invade through the corneal epithelium and sclera into the anterior chamber and through the soft tissues into the orbit. Thus, it is often necessary to remove a thin lamella of the cornea or sclera to achieve tumor-free margins and to decrease the chance for tumor recurrence. The management of limbal lesions could involve alcohol epitheliectomy or corneal epitheliectomy with a beaver blade for the corneal component and partial lamellar scleroconjunctivectomy with wide margins for the conjunctival component followed by freeze–thaw cryotherapy to the remaining adjacent bulbar conjunctiva. Bowman's layer should be respected because its removal would facilitate the intraocular penetration of any recurrence [43, 44].

In all cases, the full conjunctival component along with the underlying Tenon's fascia should be excised totally. Those tumors in the forniceal region can be managed by wide local resection and cryotherapy. In diffuse and extended lesions where complete resection is difficult, the largest possible extirpation must be made which must also allow for a precise histopathological diagnostic.

Because cells from these friable tumors can seed into adjacent tissues, a gentle technique without touching the tumor (no-touch technique) is advised. Additionally, the operative field should be left dry to minimize the seeding of cells. In some cases, microscopically controlled excision (Mohs surgery) is performed at the time of surgery to ensure tumor-free margins [45].

7.1.1.1 Incisional biopsy

An extensive suspicious tumor that is symptomatic or suspected to be malignant can be approached by incisional wedge biopsy or punch biopsy. In general, it should be concerned if tumors occupy 4 clock hours or less on the bulbar conjunctiva, excisional biopsy is preferable to incisional biopsy. Incisional biopsy is also appropriate for lesions that are ideally treated with radiotherapy, chemotherapy, or other topical medications. These include metastatic tumors, and some cases of squamous cell carcinoma that are unsuitable for surgical management [44].

7.1.1.2 Excisional biopsy

Primary excisional biopsy is appropriate for relatively smaller tumors (≦4 clock hours limbal tumor or≦15 mm basal dimension) that are symptomatic or suspected to be malignant. In these situations, excisional biopsy is preferred over incisional biopsy to avoid inadvertent tumor seeding [44].

7.1.2 Eyelid SCC treatment

Surgery remains the main modality for the management of periocular cancer. Unlike other treatment modalities, it allows histological confirmation of the diagnosis. Furthermore, examination of the excision margin assesses the adequacy of tumor clearance. To minimize the risk of incomplete excision, the larger safe margin of excision with at least 4–6 mm for SCC was recommended [46, 47].

Margin control can be achieved using frozen sections, but there are inherent inaccuracies in frozen-section techniques, and it is not unusual for frozen sections to be clear with involved margins on paraffin-fixed specimens. Confirmation of tumor clearance is essential before undertaking periocular reconstruction. Routine paraffin fixed specimens take several days to be processed, but the specimens can be processed within 24–48 h by prior arrangement with the local pathologist, allowing delayed reconstruction.

As it allows three-dimensional assessment of the tumor margins, Mos micrographic surgery (MMS) has excellent cure rates for non-melanoma skin cancers and is widely regarded as the gold standard for tumor excision [27].

Supplemental cryotherapy, topical chemotherapy and irradiation should be applied if the tumor margin is unclear or if there is residual involvement of bulbar conjunctiva.

7.1.3 Reconstruction after surgical excision

Eyelid or periocular malignancies require different considerations from other cutaneous malignancies of the same pathohistological cell type. It needs unique anatomic considerations to preserve the functional impact of ocular protection and vision after wide excision and reconstruction.

For a small conjunctival lesion, double layers closure with Tenon's fascia first and then conjunctiva over wound by primary suture may be enough. In cases where excessive conjunctiva is sacrificed, autologous conjunctival or buccal mucosa grafts, or amniotic membrane graft may be employed for reconstruction. For eyelid lesion, the primary suture is suitable for a small lesion, but an autologous graft or rotational flap may be needed for the extensive lesion.

7.2 Topical adjuvating treatments

Mitomycin C (MMC) is an antineoplastic and antibiotic agent. 5-fluorouracil (5FU) is an anticancer drug that interrupts DNA replication and cell growth. These agents are often used by an ophthalmologist in glaucoma and pterygium surgery to prevent inappropriate scar formation, especially MMC.

In cases with positive margins related to inadequate surgical excision, extensive tumors, higher recurrence, or more local invasion especially those with the extensive corneal component, treatment with topical MMC, 5FU, or interferon α (IFNα) and interferon 2b (IFN2b) as an adjuvant after surgical removal have been employed [48–51].

Topical chemotherapy enables to treat the entire ocular surface and is not dependent upon surgical margins. It may be preferred as primary treatment over the surgery by some patients who are inadequate to surgery or refuse surgery.

Subconjunctival and perilesional injections to treat OSSN have also been proposed, however, the evidence is limited and requires more studies [52].

In general, the adverse effects are minimal and tolerance in 5FU and IFN. The ocular surface toxicity and other serious adverse effects are much greater in MMC than in 5FU or IFN-b. It is the main drawback of MMC. To relieve the side effects, preservative-free artificial tears, or short-term use of the topical steroid to minimize ocular surface irritation could be used as needed. Applying petroleum jelly to the lower eyelid skin is recommended to reduce skin irritation and toxicity. Additionally, it may be instructed to occlude the punctum briefly after applying the medication to minimize the risk of punctal stenosis [53].

7.2.1 Mitomycin C (MMC)

Using topical 0.02–0.04% MMC eyedrops are very effective which show high-resolution rates ranging from 76–100% and low recurrence rates ranging from 0–20% [54–58]. Alvarez had recommended MMC in 4 week cycles of 0.04% four times a day for 1 week, followed by 3 weeks of no treatment, with cycles repeated until resolution [53]. Others may use MMC with shorter breaks, such as topically 4 times daily for a 1-week period followed by a 1-week hiatus to allow the ocular surface to recover, and this cycle is repeated once again.

Its propensity for causing ocular surface toxicity and other serious adverse effects is much greater than 5FU or IFN-b. These include allergy, itching, pain, conjunctival hyperaemia, punctate staining of the cornea, punctal stenosis corneal-scleral melting, disturbance of tear film stability, goblet cell loss, squamous metaplasia and limbal stem cells deficiency [53, 59–61].

Chemoreduction with topical MMC followed by interferon alfa 2b (1 million IU/mL) 4 times daily, or topical Cyclosporine A (0,05%) combined with a topical low dose of MMC (0,01%) had also been prescribed as the effective treatments in extensive CIN cases where surgical resection with safety margins is infeasible and corneal extension resection and the repetitive cycles of MMC adjunctive could cause a depletion of limbal stem cells and other commented side effects on the ocular surface [62].

7.2.2 5-fluorouracil (5FU)

1% of 5FU used as topical eye-drops shows very effective in treating OSSN with high-resolution rates of 82–100% and low recurrence rates of 10–14% [58, 62–65].

It is recommended four times a day for 1 week, and then stop the drug for 3 weeks. This protocol could continue until resolution [62–64].

Side effects of 5FU are generally mild and well-tolerated. These may include pain, tearing, redness, eyelid edema and keratopathy [63]. It is reported that short-term complications include lid toxicity in 52% of patients, keratopathy in 11% and epiphora in 5% [66].

7.2.3 Interferon (IFN α-2b)

IFN can be used as topical eye-drops, subconjunctival perilesional injections, or both [67, 68]. Both forms have shown great success in treating OSSN.

In cases of CIN, the combination of subconjunctival and topical treatment of IFN α-2b showed the average time to complete tumor response at mean of 5.5 weeks (range 2–12). For INF α-2b topical treatment, the average time to complete tumor response is 11 weeks (range 2–59). Injection treatment had the benefit of rapid tumor resolution [67].

Topical IFN α-2b, 1 million IU/ ml, four times daily, until resolution following with at least 1–3 months have been recommended. Weekly subconjunvtival injection of 3 million IU in 0.5ml of IFN α-2b until tumor resolution is an alternative [69].

The resolution rates showed 81–100% in topical administration and 87–100% in injections [68, 70–72]. IFN eye-drops also have remarkably low recurrence rates ranging from 0–4% [58, 71, 72].

Topical IFN eye-drops are very well tolerated by patients and nearly without side effects or discomfortable. Some follicular conjunctivitis was found [71]. Injections of IFN are also well-tolerated, but patients typically experience mild flu-like symptoms for about 24 hours following the injection [71].

7.3 Cryotherapy

Intraoperative cryotherapy by a double freeze-slow thaw method applied on conjunctival margins of the excised area has proved to diminish recurrences significantly after surgical excision in pre-cancerous and SCC in situ, but not suitable for invasive cancers [73].

The advantages of cryotherapy include the elimination of subclinical or microscopic malignant tumor cells and the prevention of recurrence. The adverse effects include conjunctival chemosis, cataract formation, uveitis, thinning scleral and corneal. Frozen globe and risk of phthisis bulbi could unexpectedly develop if cryotherapy had been excessively used [74].

It is also safe and useful for cutaneous SCC in situ in patients who refuse surgery, poor surgical candidates or with bleeding disorders.

7.4 Radiation therapy

Radiotherapeutic treatment has been limited to brachytherapy techniques either alone for whom surgery is risky, or as adjuvant therapy after surgical resection for whom the disease has spread to nerves/lymph nodes or with poorly defined margins.

When conjunctival SCC invades deeply into the sclera or into the globe, topical chemotherapeutic agents and cryotherapy might be ineffective due to not penetrating the sclera or into the eye, and enucleation is often necessary [68, 75]. To preserve vision and salvage eyeball, plaque radiotherapy had been reported as reliable alternative treatment without globe removal for conjunctival SCC demonstrating scleral invasion and/or intraocular involvement.

Using Beta radiation with strontium-90 source as adjunctive therapy to control residual microscopic tumor following surgical resection of conjunctival SCC had been reported. It revealed excellent control rates with only 3 in total 131 patients indicating recurrent after a 30-Gy dose [76], Similar results have been observed with ruthenium-106 after a total 320-Gy dose delivered at the surface without recurrence at 22 months [77]. Gamma radiotherapy using I125 has also been explored as an adjunctive treatment to excision for invasive conjunctival SCC because it has a deeper penetrability compared with beta radiation [78].

Arepalli and Shields had explored an alternative to enucleation using plaque radiotherapy with a gamma source of I125 for invasive conjunctival SCC. Plaque radiotherapy can be an effective alternative to enucleation for residual scleral-invasive conjunctival SCC following resection. In final, total globe salvage was achieved in 10 cases from their total 15 SCC patients with scleral (all cases) and anterior chamber invasion (3 cases). However, 4 cases showed further distant conjunctival tumor recurrence (remote of the radiotherapy site) with orbital involvement at 5 months after plaque radiotherapy, necessitating enucleation (n = 2) or orbital exenteration (n = 2). Complications included cataract (n = 13), iris telangiectasia (n = 5), corneal epithelial defect (n = 4), corneal edema (n = 3), and glaucoma (n = 1). One patient required enucleation due to a nonhealing epithelial defect and chronic ocular irritation [79].

In the management of eyelid malignancies, adjuvant radiotherapy has been recommended for eyelid malignancies with aggressive histologic subtype, perineural invasion, or nodal metastasis at presentation [80]. Radiotherapy is used as an adjunct to surgery in cases of incomplete tumor excision and/or perineural invasion [81, 82]. Although, radiotherapy alone is also an alternative to surgery for patients who are not candidates for surgery, there are several drawbacks. The recurrence rates are higher after radiotherapy alone than surgery [83]. Furthermore, when recurrence occurs, it is usually difficult to manage and definitively diagnose [84]. Unlike surgery, radiation therapy does not readily demonstrate histological evidence of tumor clearance. It is also noted that a large dose of radiotherapy may cause ocular complications leading to visual disturbance.

7.5 Chemotherapy

Systemic chemotherapy is recommended for patients in the advanced stage with distant metastasis and can be considered for patients with extensive nodal disease.

7.6 Other treatment modalities

Other treatment modalities currently with favorable outcomes include radiotherapy, surgical excision in combination with absolute alcohol, vitamin A, excimer laser, topical imiquimod 5% cream, and adjuvant topical or perilesional chemotherapy [50].

7.7 Management of Intraocular or/and infraorbital invasion

Orbital invasion by eyelid SCC occurs in 4–8% of cases [7, 27]. Conjunctival SCC can represent 0 ~ 13% of intraocular and/or 1–6% of orbital local invasion. The orbital invasion should be suspected if a patient with a current or previously treated periocular malignancy presents with a palpable orbital mass, globe displacement, limitation of eye movement, numbness, or pain in the distribution of the trigeminal nerve (**Figure 6**) [85, 86]. If Intraocular or/and infraorbital invasion occurs, it has devastating visual consequences [32, 33, 35].

The intraocular spread tends to follow recurrence of the conjunctival lesion after attempted excision. Modes of invasion may include direct invasion through the sclera, along the tract of the anterior ciliary vessels, or inoculation through intraocular surgery incision [87].

Although, there have been reports of local control achieved with globe-sparing surgeries [79, 88], enucleation or exenteration is usually required to manage intraocular or/and intra-orbital invasion with or without adjunctive radiotherapy.

Local tumor clearance is usually possible by orbital exenteration with or without adjunctive radiotherapy. However, the perineural invasion occurs commonly in such cases, and increases the risk of incomplete excision even after exenteration [85]. Furthermore, perineural invasion worsens the prognosis because of extensive orbital, and sometimes intracranial involvement. A meta-analysis of 9 publications on large series of exenterations between 1954 and 2005 indicated that 89/559 (16%) cases were for conjunctival SCC and required exenteration for advanced disease [89].

Orbital exenteration rates are 6% at 5 years in the US, but are higher in HIV endemic areas, with 13/23 cases (56%) reported in a case series in Zimbabwe [33]. Risk factors predictive of orbital exenteration were positive margins at primary resection, perineural invasion, positive nodal status, and medial canthal tumor location [89].

7.8 Target therapy

The discovery of overexpression of the epidermal growth factor receptor (EGFR, a transmembrane tyrosine kinase receptor in the ErbB family) in SCC has opened the door to consideration of targeted therapy in inoperable cases of advanced BCC or cutaneous SCC of the orbit and periocular region [90].

Recently, both Yin's group and El-Sawy's group show successful outcomes after oral erlotinib (EGFR inhibitor) treatment in some patients who have advanced SCC with orbital invasion and regional lymph nodes metastasis [91, 92]. However, several reports also show that patients often acquire resistance. Several publications point out that despite EGFR inhibition, there are multiple downstream signaling pathways that serve as alternatives and that are found to be persistently activated, thus permitting cancer resistance to EGFR-inhibitors [93, 94]. Additionally, less than 5% of head and neck cancers contain EGFR mutations, which may partially explain the limited efficacy in using EGFR inhibitors and the current lack of FDA-approved for HNSCC [93, 95]. For the efficacy of EGFR inhibitor in the treatment of cutaneous SCC, more studies are needed to further conform.

In 2018, designated by the FDA as a breakthrough therapy, cemiplimab-rwlc, a PD-1–blocking antibody, became the first drug to receive FDA approval for the treatment of patients with advanced cutaneous SCC. Of the 75 patients with metastatic CSCC, 46.7% achieved an objective response; of the 33 patients with locally advanced CSCC, 48.5% achieved an objective response. Furthermore, 60% of patients with metastatic CSCC and 63% of patients with locally advanced CSCC maintained a response to treatment for ≥6 months [96].

With the Libtayo approval, the FDA has approved six immune checkpoint inhibitors targeting the PD-1/PD-L1 pathway for treating a variety of tumors, from the bladder to head and neck cancer, and now advanced cutaneous squamous-cell carcinoma.

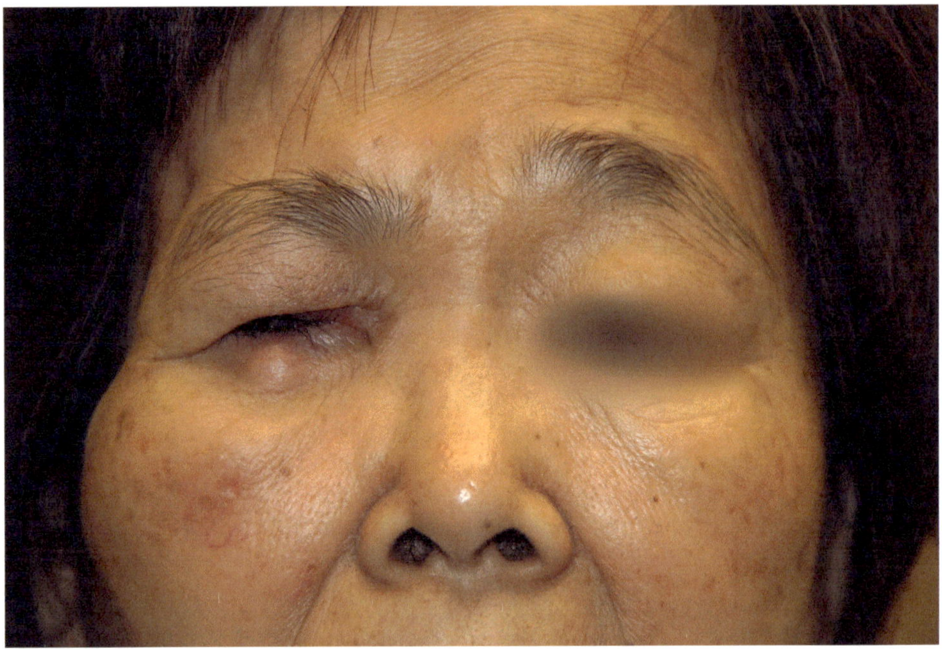

Figure 6.
A patient with squamous cell carcinoma of the right eyelid with orbital metastasis: Periocular mass, proptosis, facial numbness and palsy.

8. Regional lymph nodes and distant organ metastasis

Early diagnosis and adequate treatment of the eyelid SCC is very important, because of its ability to invade the orbital and intracranial legions and metastasis to the lymph nodes and distant organs. Regional lymph nodes are generally believed to be the most common first site of metastasis for SCC of the eyelid. The incidence of regional lymph node metastasis of eyelid SCC varies widely from 10% to 24.3% [97]. with most regional metastases occurring in the parotid, preauricular, and submandibular nodes. Distant metastasis is much less common, reported in 6.2% of cases [28].

Radical dissection with sentinel lymph node biopsy for patients with extensive lesions especially with perineurial invasion and recurrent lesions may get benefit if there is a ruling out distant metastasis. A high degree of suspicion for the orbital invasion along sensory nerves should be maintained. Perineural spread of cutaneous SCC is associated with an increased risk of local recurrence and distant metastasis, but may also be the direct cause of death when the primary tumor on the head and face gains access to the intracranial cavity via the cranial nerves [98, 99]. Risk factors have been found to correlate with the increased death and poor prognosis for cutaneous SCC, including prior treatments, lesion size ≥2 cm, increased depth, poor histopathological differentiation and immunosuppression [100]. In Nasser's study, patients who had a lymph node metastasis at presentation or during follow-up had tumors that were stage T2C (according to AJCC, 9th edition; or T2b in AJCC, 8th edition) or higher at and ≥ 18 mm in greatest dimension at presentation. This finding will help practitioners select patients for closer surveillance for nodal metastasis or possibly for SLN biopsy [101].

9. Recurrence

Recurrence rates in OSCC range from 5–50% [33, 102–105]. Galor et al. found that the 1-year recurrence rate was 10% and the 5-year recurrence rate was 21%, with a mean time to recurrence of 2.5 years when analyzing 389 excised OSSN lesions [73]. In Savino's study, the overall recurrence rate was significantly higher (64%) in their advanced ocular surface squamous cell carcinoma (OSSC, T3 and T4 stage) cases series after long-term follow-up (median: 31 months, range: 6–120 months) [106].

In advanced, OSCC involving periocular tissues and/or orbit is an aggressive disease with a high recurrence rate. Multicentric disease, positive surgical margins, inferior tarsus localization, and surgery without adjuvant therapies are strong predictors of recurrence and are the main factors affecting prognosis [105].

The type of treatment is also correlated with the recurrence rate. Sudesh et al. reported a recurrence rate of 28.5% with surgical excision alone and 7.7% with surgical excision and cryotherapy [107]. Adjuvant topical therapy showed effectiveness in decreasing recurrence rates, particularly in patients with positive margins, histological high-risk SCC, tarsal, and multicentric pattern anatomical involvement [73, 108].

The presence of positive margins can increase the risk of recurrence by as much as 10-fold, from 5–50% [35].

The microscopic and histologic information of cutaneous and periocular SCC is helpful to evaluate the recurrence, perineural invasion, local invasion, and metastasis. Histological well-differentiated tumors are associated with a lower risk of subclinical tumor extension, recurrence, and orbital invasion [27, 100]. Histologic specimens should be carefully examined for evidence of perineural invasion when facing cases of particularly aggressive tumors or in patients with symptoms of trigeminal pain, trigeminal-distribution sensory deficit, facial palsy, orbital pain, or biopsy of the supraorbital orbital nerve [28, 109]. Perineural invasion is associated with high local invasion, recurrence, and distant metastasis [98–99].

The local recurrence rates for SCC range from 2.4% to 36.9% at 5 years [7, 28]. The perineural invasion has been found to be present in approximately 8–14% of cases of facial and periorbital SCC [7, 110].

10. Conclusions

Squamous cell carcinoma of the eyelid and ocular surface is an aggressive malignancy and maybe vision- and life-threatening although it grows slowly. Precise diagnosis along with appropriate management is a prerequisite.

Conflict of interest

The authors declare no conflict of interest.

Author details

Jin-Jhe Wang[1,2], Yueh-Ju Tsai[2,3] and Chau-Yin Chen[1,2,4]*

1 Department of Ophthalmology, Chiayi Chang Gung Memorial Hospital, Chiayi, Taiwan

2 College of Medicine, Chang Gung University, Taoyuan, Taiwan

3 Department of Ophthalmology, Chang Gung Memorial Hospital, Taoyuan, Taiwan

4 Department of Nursing, Chang Gung University of Science and Technology, Chiayi, Taiwan

*Address all correspondence to: ccy423@gmail.com

References

[1] Mehta M, Fay A. Squamous cell carcinoma of the eyelid and conjunctiva. International Ophthalmology Clinics. 2009;**49**(1):111-121

[2] Gallagher RP, Ma B, McLean DI, et al. Trends in basal cell carcinoma, squamous cell carcinoma, and melanoma of the skin from 1973 through 1987. Journal of the American Academy of Dermatology. 1990;**23**(3 Pt 1):413-421

[3] Wawrzynski J, Tudge I, Fitzgerald E, et al. Report on the incidence of squamous cell carcinomas affecting the eyelids in England over a 15-year period (2000-2014). The British Journal of Ophthalmology. 2018;**102**(10):1358-1361

[4] Deprez M, Uffer S. Clinicopathological features of eyelid skin tumors. A retrospective study of 5504 cases and review of literature. The American Journal of Dermatopathology. 2009;**31**(3):256-262

[5] Limawararut V, Leibovitch I, Sullivan T, Selva D. Periocular squamous cell carcinoma. Clinical & Experimental Ophthalmology. 2007;**35**(2):174-185

[6] Cook BE Jr, Bartley GB. Epidemiologic characteristics and clinical course of patients with malignant eyelid tumors in an incidence cohort in Olmsted County, Minnesota. Ophthalmology. 1999;**106**(4):746-750

[7] Donaldson MJ, Sullivan TJ, Whitehead KJ, Williamson RM. Squamous cell carcinoma of the eyelids. The British Journal of Ophthalmology. 2002;**86**(10):1161-1165

[8] Shields CL, Alset AE, Boal NS, et al. Conjunctival Tumors in 5002 cases. Comparative analysis of benign versus malignant counterparts. The 2016 James D. Allen lecture. American Journal of Ophthalmology. 2017;**173**:106-133

[9] Sun EC, Fears TR, Goedert JJ. Epidemiology of squamous cell conjunctival cancer. Cancer Epidemiology, Biomarkers & Prevention. 1997;**6**(2):73-77

[10] Lee GA, Hirst LW. Incidence of ocular surface epithelial dysplasia in metropolitan Brisbane. A 10-year survey. Archives of Ophthalmology. 1992;**110**(4):525-527

[11] Ramberg I, Toft PB, Heegaard S. Carcinomas of the lacrimal drainage system. Survey of Ophthalmology. 2020;**65**(6):691-707

[12] Koturović Z, Knežević M, Rašić DM. Clinical significance of routine lacrimal sac biopsy during dacryocystorhinostomy: A comprehensive review of literature. Bosnian Journal of Basic Medical Sciences. 2017;**17**(1):1-8

[13] Newton R, Ferlay J, Reeves G, Beral V, Parkin DM. Effect of ambient solar ultraviolet radiation on incidence of squamous-cell carcinoma of the eye. Lancet. 1996;**347**(9013):1450-1451

[14] Green AC, Olsen CM. Cutaneous squamous cell carcinoma: an epidemiological review. The British Journal of Dermatology. 2017;**177**(2):373-381

[15] Scotto J, Kopf AW, Urbach F. Non-melanoma skin cancer among Caucasians in four areas of the United States. Cancer. 1974;**34**(4):1333-1338

[16] Garrett GL, Blanc PD, Boscardin J, et al. Incidence of and risk factors for skin cancer in organ transplant recipients

in the United States. JAMA Dermatology. 2017;**153**(3):296-303

[17] Omland SH, Ahlström MG, Gerstoft J, et al. Risk of skin cancer in patients with HIV: A Danish nationwide cohort study. Journal of the American Academy of Dermatology. 2018;**79**(4):689-695

[18] Fania L, Abeni D, Esposito I, et al. Behavioral and demographic factors associated with occurrence of non-melanoma skin cancer in organ transplant recipients. Giornale Italiano di Dermatologia e Venereologia. 2020;**155**(5):669-675

[19] Stewart WB, Nicholson DH, Hamilton G, Tenzel RR, Spencer WH. Eyelid tumors anmd renal transplantation. Archives of Ophthalmology. 1980;**98**(10): 1771-1772

[20] Kraemer KH, Lee MM, Scotto J. Xeroderma pigmentosum. Cutaneous, ocular, and neurologic abnormalities in 830 published cases. Archives of Dermatology. 1987;**123**(2):241-250

[21] Alam M, Ratner D. Cutaneous squamous-cell carcinoma. The New England Journal of Medicine. 2001;**344**(13):975-983

[22] Di Girolamo N, Atik A, McCluskey PJ, Wakefield D. Matrix metalloproteinases and their inhibitors in squamous cell carcinoma of the conjunctiva. The Ocular Surface. 2013;**11**(3):193-205

[23] Wang JJ, Lee KF, Chen CY. Collision tumor of sebaceous carcinoma and squamous cell carcinoma of the eyelid: Case report. European Journal of Ophthalmology. 2021. Advance Online Publication. DOI: 10.1177/11206721211016303

[24] Cassarino DS, Derienzo DP, Barr RJ. Cutaneous squamous cell carcinoma: a comprehensive clinicopathologic classification. Part one. Journal of Cutaneous Pathology. 2006;**33**(3):191-206

[25] Jakobiec FA, Mendoza PR. Eyelid sebaceous carcinoma: Clinicopathologic and multiparametric immunohistochemical analysis that includes adipophilin. American Journal of Ophthalmology. 2014;**157**(1):186-208.e2

[26] Kersten RC, Ewing-Chow D, Kulwin DR, Gallon M. Accuracy of clinical diagnosis of cutaneous eyelid lesions. Ophthalmology. 1997;**104**(3):479-484

[27] Malhotra R, Huilgol SC, Huynh NT, Selva D. The Australian Mohs database: Periocular squamous cell carcinoma. Ophthalmology. 2004;**111**(4):617-623

[28] Faustina M, Diba R, Ahmadi MA, Esmaeli B. Patterns of regional and distant metastasis in patients with eyelid and periocular squamous cell carcinoma. Ophthalmology. 2004;**111**(10):1930-1932

[29] Sullivan TJ. Squamous cell carcinoma of eyelid, periocular, and periorbital skin. International Ophthalmology Clinics. 2009;**49**(4):17-24

[30] Shields CL, Shields JA. Tumors of the conjunctiva and cornea. Indian Journal of Ophthalmology. 2019;**67**(12):1930-1948

[31] Yanoff M, Duker JS. Eyelid Malignancies. In: Vaughn GJ, Dortzbach RK, Gayre GS, editors. Ophthalmology. 4th ed. Edinburgh: Mosby Elsevier; 2014. p. 1038

[32] Cervantes G, Rodríguez AA Jr, Leal AG. Squamous cell carcinoma of the conjunctiva: Clinicopathological features in 287 cases. Canadian Journal of Ophthalmology. 2002;**37**(1):14-20

[33] Tunc M, Char DH, Crawford B, Miller T. Intraepithelial and invasive squamous cell carcinoma of the conjunctiva: Analysis of 60 cases. The British Journal of Ophthalmology. 1999;**83**(1):98-103

[34] Chen CY, Wang SW, Lai CH, Chuang HC, Lin YY, Wang JJ. The clinical presentation and treatment of an invasive conjunctival squamous spindle cell carcinoma. Taiwan Journal of Ophthalmology. 2021. Advance Online Publication. DOI: 10.4103/tjo.tjo_26_21

[35] Erie JC, Campbell RJ, Liesegang TJ. Conjunctival and corneal intraepithelial and invasive neoplasia. Ophthalmology. 1986;**93**(2):176-183

[36] Iliff WJ, Marback R, Green WR. Invasive squamous cell carcinoma of the conjunctiva. Archives of Ophthalmology. 1975;**93**(2):119-122

[37] Johnson TE, Tabbara KF, Weatherhead RG, Kersten RC, Rice C, Nasr AM. Secondary squamous cell carcinoma of the orbit. Archives of Ophthalmology. 1997;**115**(1):75-78

[38] Krishna Y, Coupland SE. Lacrimal sac Tumors--a review. Asia-Pacific journal of ophthalmology (Philadelphia, Pa.). 2017;**6**(2):173-178

[39] Song X, Wang S, Wang J, et al. Clinical management and outcomes of lacrimal sac squamous cell carcinoma. Head & Neck. 2019;**41**(4):974-981

[40] Pfeiffer ML, Savar A, Esmaeli B. Sentinel lymph node biopsy for eyelid and conjunctival tumors: What have we learned in the past decade? Ophthalmic Plastic & Reconstructive Surgery. 2013;**29**(1):57-62

[41] Shields JA, Shields CL. Management of conjunctival tumors. In: Shields JA, Shields CL, editors. Atlas of Eyelid and Conjunctival Tumors. Philadelphia: PA, Lippincott Williams and Wilkins Co; 1999. pp. 332-479

[42] Shields JA, Shields CL, De Potter P. Surgical management of circumscribed conjunctival melanomas. Ophthalmic Plastic & Reconstructive Surgery. 1998;**14**(3):208-215

[43] Rene C. Oculoplastic aspects of ocular oncology. Eye (London, England). 2013;**27**(2):199-207

[44] Shields CL, Shields JA. Tumors of the conjunctiva and cornea. Survey of Ophthalmology. 2004;**49**(1):3-24

[45] Buus DR, Tse DT, Folberg R, Buuns DR. Microscopically controlled excision of conjunctival squamous cell carcinoma. American Journal of Ophthalmology. 1994;**117**(1):97-102

[46] Abide JM, Nahai F, Bennett RG. The meaning of surgical margins. Plastic and Reconstructive Surgery. 1984;**73**(3):492-497

[47] Weinstein MC, Brodell RT, Bordeaux J, Honda K. The art and science of surgical margins for the dermatopathologist. The American Journal of Dermatopathology. 2012;**34**(7):737-745

[48] Shields CL, Demirci H, Karatza E, Shields JA. Clinical survey of 1643 melanocytic and nonmelanocytic conjunctival tumors. Ophthalmology. 2004;**111**(9):1747-1754

[49] Al Bayyat G, Arreaza-Kaufman D, Venkateswaran N, Galor A, Karp CL. Update on pharmacotherapy for ocular surface squamous neoplasia. Eye and Vision (London). 2019;**6**:24

[50] Miller CV, Wolf A, Klingenstein A, et al. Clinical outcome of advanced

squamous cell carcinoma of the conjunctiva. Eye (London, England). 2014;**28**(8):962-967

[51] Rootman DB, McGowan HD, Yücel YH, Pavlin CJ, Simpson ER. Intraocular extension of conjunctival invasive squamous cell carcinoma after pterygium surgery and cataract extraction. Eye & Contact Lens. 2012;**38**(2):133-136

[52] Sun Y, Hua R. Long-term efficacy and safety of subconjunctival/perilesional 5-fluorouracil injections for ocular surface squamous neoplasia. Drug Design, Development and Therapy. 2020;**14**:5659-5665

[53] Alvarez OP, Zein M, Galor A, Karp CL. Management of ocular surface squamous neoplasia: Bowman Club lecture 2021. BMJ Open Ophthalmology. 2021;**6**(1):e000842

[54] Ballalai PL, Erwenne CM, Martins MC, Lowen MS, Barros JN. Long-term results of topical mitomycin C 0.02% for primary and recurrent conjunctival-corneal intraepithelial neoplasia. Ophthalmic. Plastic and Reconstructive Surgery. 2009;**25**(4):296-299

[55] Frucht-Pery J, Sugar J, Baum J, et al. Mitomycin C treatment for conjunctival-corneal intraepithelial neoplasia: A multicenter experience. Ophthalmology. 1997;**104**(12):2085-2093

[56] Hirst LW. Randomized controlled trial of topical mitomycin C for ocular surface squamous neoplasia: Early resolution. Ophthalmology. 2007;**114**(5):976-982

[57] Prabhasawat P, Tarinvorakup P, Tesavibul N, et al. Topical 0.002% mitomycin C for the treatment of conjunctival-corneal intraepithelial neoplasia and squamous cell carcinoma. Cornea. 2005;**24**(4):443-448

[58] Kusumesh R, Ambastha A, Kumar S, Sinha BP, Imam N. Retrospective comparative study of topical interferon α2b versus mitomycin C for primary ocular surface squamous neoplasia. Cornea. 2017;**36**(3):327-331

[59] Dogru M, Erturk H, Shimazaki J, Tsubota K, Gul M. Tear function and ocular surface changes with topical mitomycin (MMC) treatment for primary corneal intraepithelial neoplasia. Cornea. 2003;**22**(7):627-639

[60] Dudney BW, Malecha MA. Limbal stem cell deficiency following topical mitomycin C treatment of conjunctival-corneal intraepithelial neoplasia. American Journal of Ophthalmology. 2004;**137**(5):950-951

[61] Khong JJ, Muecke J. Complications of mitomycin C therapy in 100 eyes with ocular surface neoplasia. The British Journal of Ophthalmology. 2006;**90**(7):819-822

[62] Huerva V, Mateo AJ, Mangues I, Jurjo C. Short-term mitomycin C followed by long-term interferon alpha2beta for conjunctiva-cornea intraepithelial neoplasia. Cornea. 2006;**25**(10):1220-1223

[63] Parrozzani R, Frizziero L, Trainiti S, et al. Topical 1% 5-fluoruracil as a sole treatment of corneoconjunctival ocular surface squamous neoplasia: Long-term study. The British Journal of Ophthalmology. 2017;**101**(8):1094-1099

[64] Venkateswaran N, Mercado C, Galor A, Karp CL. Comparison of topical 5-fluorouracil and interferon alfa-2b as primary treatment modalities for ocular surface squamous neoplasia. American Journal of Ophthalmology. 2019;**199**:216-222

[65] Joag MG, Sise A, Murillo JC, et al. Topical 5-fluorouracil 1% as primary treatment for ocular surface squamous neoplasia. Ophthalmology. 2016;**123**(7):1442-1448

[66] Rudkin AK, Dodd T, Muecke JS. The differential diagnosis of localised amelanotic limbal lesions: A review of 162 consecutive excisions. The British Journal of Ophthalmology. 2011;**95**(3):350-354

[67] Huerva V, Mangues I. Treatment of conjunctival squamous neoplasias with interferon alpha 2ab. Journal Français d'Ophtalmologie. 2008;**31**(3):317-325

[68] Karp CL, Galor A, Chhabra S, Barnes SD, Alfonso EC. Subconjunctival/perilesional recombinant interferon α2b for ocular surface squamous neoplasia: A 10-year review. Ophthalmology. 2010;**117**(12):2241-2246

[69] Vann RR, Karp CL. Perilesional and topical interferon alfa-2b for conjunctival and corneal neoplasia. Ophthalmology. 1999;**106**(1):91-97

[70] Shields CL, Kaliki S, Kim HJ, et al. Interferon for ocular surface squamous neoplasia in 81 cases: Outcomes based on the American joint committee on cancer classification. Cornea. 2013;**32**(3):248-256

[71] Kusumesh R, Ambastha A, Sinha B, Kumar R. Topical interferon α-2b as a single therapy for primary ocular surface squamous neoplasia. Asia-Pacific journal of ophthalmology (Philadelphia, Pa.). 2015;**4**(5):279-282

[72] Shields CL, Constantinescu AB, Paulose SA, et al. Primary treatment of ocular surface squamous neoplasia with topical interferon alpha-2b: Comparative analysis of outcomes based on original tumor configuration. Indian Journal of Ophthalmology. 2021;**69**(3):563-567

[73] Galor A, Karp CL, Oellers P, et al. Predictors of ocular surface squamous neoplasia recurrence after excisional surgery. Ophthalmology. 2012;**119**(10):1974-1981

[74] Eichler MD, Fraunfelder FT. Cryotherapy for conjunctival lymphoid tumors. American Journal of Ophthalmology. 1994;**118**(4):463-467

[75] Al-Barrag A, Al-Shaer M, Al-Matary N, Al-Hamdani M. 5-fluorouracil for the treatment of intraepithelial neoplasia and squamous cell carcinoma of the conjunctiva, and cornea. Clinical Ophthalmology. 2010;**4**:801-808

[76] Kearsley JH, Fitchew RS, Taylor RG. Adjunctive radiotherapy with strontium-90 in the treatment of conjunctival squamous cell carcinoma. International Journal of Radiation Oncology, Biology, Physics. 1988;**14**(3):435-443

[77] Zehetmayer M, Menapace R, Kulnig W. Combined local excision and brachytherapy with ruthenium-106 in the treatment of epibulbar malignancies. Ophthalmologica. 1993;**207**(3):133-139

[78] Walsh-Conway N, Conway RM. Plaque brachytherapy for the management of ocular surface malignancies with corneoscleral invasion. Clinical & Experimental Ophthalmology. 2009;**37**(6):577-583

[79] Arepalli S, Kaliki S, Shields CL, Emrich J, Komarnicky L, Shields JA. Plaque radiotherapy in the management of scleral-invasive conjunctival squamous cell carcinoma: An analysis of 15 eyes. JAMA Ophthalmology. 2014;**132**(6):691-696

[80] Hsu A, Frank SJ, Ballo MT, et al. Postoperative adjuvant external-beam radiation therapy for cancers of the eyelid and conjunctiva. Ophthalmic Plastic & Reconstructive Surgery. 2008;**24**(6):444-449

[81] Murchison AP, Walrath JD, Washington CV. Non-surgical treatments of primary, non-melanoma eyelid malignancies: A review. Clinical & Experimental Ophthalmology. 2011;**39**(1):65-93

[82] Schlienger P, Brunin F, Desjardins L, Laurent M, Haye C, Vilcoq JR. External radiotherapy for carcinoma of the eyelid: Report of 850 cases treated. International Journal of Radiation Oncology, Biology, Physics. 1996;**34**(2):277-287

[83] Fitzpatrick PJ, Thompson GA, Easterbrook WM, Gallie BL, Payne DG. Basal and squamous cell carcinoma of the eyelids and their treatment by radiotherapy. International Journal of Radiation Oncology, Biology, Physics. 1984;**10**(4):449-454

[84] Leatherbarrow B. Oculoplastic Surgery. 2nd ed. London: Informa Healthcare; 2011

[85] Leibovitch I, McNab A, Sullivan T, Davis G, Selva D. Orbital invasion by periocular basal cell carcinoma. Ophthalmology. 2005;**112**(4):717-723

[86] Tyers AG. Orbital exenteration for invasive skin tumours. Eye (London, England). 2006;**20**(10):1165-1170

[87] Shields JA, Shields CL, De Potter P. Surgical management of conjunctival tumors. The 1994 Lynn B. McMahan lecture. Archives of Ophthalmology. 1997;**115**(6):808-815

[88] Char DH, Crawford JB, Howes EL Jr, Weinstein AJ. Resection of intraocular squamous cell carcinoma. The British Journal of Ophthalmology. 1992;**76**(2):123-125

[89] Ben Simon GJ, Schwarcz RM, Douglas R, Fiaschetti D, McCann JD, Goldberg RA. Orbital exenteration: One size does not fit all. American Journal of Ophthalmology. 2005;**139**(1):11-17

[90] Ch'ng S, Low I, Ng D, et al. Epidermal growth factor receptor: A novel biomarker for aggressive head and neck cutaneous squamous cell carcinoma. Human Pathology. 2008;**39**(3):344-349

[91] El-Sawy T, Sabichi AL, Myers JN, et al. Epidermal growth factor receptor inhibitors for treatment of orbital squamous cell carcinoma. Archives of Ophthalmology. 2012;**130**(12): 1608-1611

[92] Yin VT, Pfeiffer ML, Esmaeli B. Targeted therapy for orbital and periocular basal cell carcinoma and squamous cell carcinoma. Ophthalmic Plastic & Reconstructive Surgery. 2013;**29**(2):87-92

[93] Rehmani HS, Issaeva N. EGFR in head and neck squamous cell carcinoma: Exploring possibilities of novel drug combinations. Annals of Translational Medicine. 2020;**8**(13):813

[94] Chen LF, Cohen EE, Grandis JR. New strategies in head and neck cancer: Understanding resistance to epidermal growth factor receptor inhibitors. Clinical Cancer Research. 2010;**16**(9):2489-2495

[95] Perisanidis C. Prevalence of EGFR tyrosine kinase domain mutations in head and neck squamous cell carcinoma: Cohort study and systematic review. In Vivo. 2017;**31**(1):23-34

[96] Libtayo (cemiplimab-rwlc) Injection [prescribing information]. Tarrytown, NY: Regeneron Pharmaceuticals; Bridgewater, NJ: sanofi-aventis U.S.; 2018

[97] Soysal HG, Markoç F. Invasive squamous cell carcinoma of the eyelids and periorbital region. The British Journal of Ophthalmology. 2007;**91**(3):325-329

[98] Wilcsek GA, Francis IC, Egan CA, Kneale KL, Sharma S, Kappagoda MB. Superior oblique palsy in a patient with a history of perineural spread from a periorbital squamous cell carcinoma. Journal of Neuro-Ophthalmology. 2000;**20**(4):240-241

[99] Veness MJ, Biankin S. Perineural spread leading to orbital invasion from skin cancer. Australasian Radiology. 2000;**44**(3):296-302

[100] Rowe DE, Carroll RJ, Day CL Jr. Prognostic factors for local recurrence, metastasis, and survival rates in squamous cell carcinoma of the skin, ear, and lip. Implications for treatment modality selection. Journal of the American Academy of Dermatology. 1992;**26**(6):976-990

[101] Nasser QJ, Roth KG, Warneke CL, Yin VT, El Sawy T, Esmaeli B. Impact of AJCC 'T' designation on risk of regional lymph node metastasis in patients with squamous carcinoma of the eyelid. The British Journal of Ophthalmology. 2014;**98**(4):498-501

[102] Cohen BH, Green WR, Iliff NT, Taxy JB, Schwab LT, de la Cruz Z. Spindle cell carcinoma of the conjunctiva. Archives of Ophthalmology. 1980;**98**(10):1809-1813

[103] Brownstein S. Mucoepidermoid carcinoma of the conjunctiva with intraocular invasion. Ophthalmology. 1981;**88**(12):1226-1230

[104] Basti S, Macsai MS. Ocular surface squamous neoplasia: A review. Cornea. 2003;**22**(7):687-704

[105] Lee GA, Hirst LW. Ocular surface squamous neoplasia. Survey of Ophthalmology. 1995;**39**(6):429-450

[106] Savino G, Cuffaro G, Maceroni M, et al. Advanced ocular surface squamous cell carcinoma (OSSC): Long-term follow-up. Graefe's Archive for Clinical and Experimental Ophthalmology. 2021;**259**(11):3437-3443

[107] Sudesh S, Rapuano CJ, Cohen EJ, Eagle RC Jr, Laibson PR. Surgical management of ocular surface squamous neoplasms: The experience from a cornea center. Cornea. 2000;**19**(3):278-283

[108] Blasi MA, Maceroni M, Sammarco MG, Pagliara MM. Mitomycin C or interferon as adjuvant therapy to surgery for ocular surface squamous neoplasia: Comparative study. European Journal of Ophthalmology. 2018;**28**(2):204-209

[109] Bowyer JD, Sullivan TJ, Whitehead KJ, Kelly LE, Allison RW. The management of perineural spread of squamous cell carcinoma to the ocular adnexae. Ophthalmic Plastic & Reconstructive Surgery. 2003;**19**(4):275-281

[110] Goepfert H, Dichtel WJ, Medina JE, Lindberg RD, Luna MD. Perineural invasion in squamous cell skin carcinoma of the head and neck. American Journal of Surgery. 1984;**148**(4):542-547

Chapter 8

Mutational Profile of Human Papilloma Virus (HPV) Induced and Non-HPV Induced Head and Neck Squamous Cell Carcinoma

Minu Jenifer Michael Raj, Fenwick Antony Edwin Rodrigues and Sivasamy Ramasamy

Abstract

Head and Neck cancer accounts for approximately 900,000 cases and over 400,000 deaths annually worldwide. The primary risk factors associated with Head and Neck cancer include usage of tobacco, alcohol consumption, Human Papillomavirus (HPV) infection and Epstein-Barr virus (EBV) infection. Few subsites of Head and Neck Squamous Cell Carcinoma (HNSCC) are associated with Human Papilloma Virus (HPV) while others remain non-associated. The anatomical, physiological, genetic, protein profile and epigenetic changes that occur in both HPV-positive and HPV-negative HNSCC has been discussed in this chapter. The mutational profile plays a crucial role in the treatment of the HNSCC patients as the HPV-positive HNSCC patients have a better prognosis compared to the HPV-negative HNSCC patients. This chapter mainly focusses on the mutational profile of both HPV-associated and non-HPV associated HNSCC tumours.

Keywords: Human Papilloma Virus (HPV), Head and Neck Squamous Cell Carcinoma (HNSCC), genes, mutations, carcinogenesis

1. Introduction

Head and Neck Squamous Cell Carcinoma (HNSCC) contribute to substantial morbidity and mortality worldwide, with an estimated 526,481 incident cases annually [1]. HNSCC arise from the mucosal epithelium of oral cavity, pharynx and larynx. Apart from the prime etiologic factors like environmental carcinogens and carcinogenic viruses, genetic predisposition plays a risk-modulating role [2] in which the large burden of mutations lead to the heterogeneity of the tumour. Human Papilloma Virus (HPV) is a well-known risk factor for malignant transformation and is increasingly associated with the majority (60–70%) of the recently diagnosed oropharyngeal cancer incidences. Majority of the HPV-induced Oropharyngeal cancers harbour high risk HPV16 primarily and to a lesser extent HPV18 and other

 IntechOpen

strains of HPV [3]. In Human papilloma virus induced tumourigenesis, HPV derived oncoproteins E6 and E7 inactivate the tumour suppressor genes p53 and pRb (retinoblastoma), resulting in the onset and eventual progression to malignancy [4]. HPV-associated HNSCC cells are poorly differentiated, non-keratinizing, and have a distinct 'basaloid' appearance in contrast to the non-HPV associated HNSCC which are usually moderately differentiated and keratinizing [5]. As the HPV DNA integrates into the host cell genome in a large proportion of HPV associated HNSCC, the tumours of HPV positive HNSCC differ at their genetic level [6]. Compared to the HPV negative HNSCC, HPV- associated HNSCCs manifest lower levels of chromosomal mutations [7]. Southern blotting, Polymerase Chain Reaction (PCR) and its variations like Reverse transcriptase and Real Time PCR, in situ hybridization, immunohistochemical staining for p16, immunostaining with anti E6, E7 antibosies, PCR in situ hybridization (PISH) are some of the techniques used for the detection of HPV in the Head and Neck cancers [8]. HPV positive HNSCC patients with lymph node metastases exhibit improved loco-regional control showing regression more quickly. They are more likely to resolve better after treatment when compared to the lymph node metastases of HPV negative HNSCC patients. Patients with HPV associated HNSCC have a better survival rate over HPV negative HNSCC patients with a 58% reduction in mortality risk [9].

2. Differences between HPV-positive and HPV-negative Head and Neck Squamous Cell Carcinoma (HNSCC)

2.1 Anatomical differences

The Head and Neck cancers arise from the tumours of mucosal epithelium in the oral cavity (lips, hard palate, buccal mucosa, floor of mouth, anterior tongue, and retromolar trigone), nasopharynx, oropharynx (palatine tonsils, lingual tonsils, soft palate, base of tongue, uvula and posterior pharyngeal wall), hypopharynx and larynx. Tumour growth in the oral cavity, hypopharynx and larynx is due to tobacco consumption and continuous alcohol abuse whereas, cancers in the pharynx (from the palatine and lingual tonsils of the oropharynx) are increasingly attributed to infection with Human Papillomavirus (HPV), primarily HPV-16, 18 and also other HPV strains. Therefore, the Head and Neck Squamous Cell Carcinoma (HNSCC) can be grouped into HPV-negative and HPV-positive [10]. The primary site of HPV-positive groups is the oropharynx (51%) and various other sites like larynx (11%), oral cavity (9%), nasopharynx (9%), and pharynx (5%) also encompass HPV positive tumours [11]. HPV is an epithelium-specific infection that does not spread though the bloodstream. Consequently, a limitation of HPV serology is that it does not specify the anatomic site of HPV infection. Hence, the elevated odds of oral cancer observed in association with oral HPV infection are considered more strong evidence for a direct relationship between HPV infection and oral cancer. The data obtained from risk factors associated with sexual behaviour, HPV exposure and oral HPV detection indicate that sexually acquired oral HPV infection is the principal risk factor for many cancers arising from the oral cavity. Based on the research findings, there is apparent evidence on the HPV transformation within the oral cavity, the tonsillar crypt epithelium, ectopic tonsillar tissue in the lateral posterior tongue or floor of mouth. This is approximated to occur in 0.4 per 100,000 individuals. These findings prove that the oral cavity is an intended site for HPV positive tumours [12, 13]. An international case-control study has estimated that HPV plays a part in approximately 3% of oral cavity cancers [14].

2.1.1 Physiological factors in HPV positive and negative HNSCC

The HPV positive HNSCC is made up of highly malignant cells that have a high nuclear to cytoplasmic ratio and exhibit little or no keratinization. These cells differ from the non-neoplastic squamous epithelium that lines the oral cavity. The HPV related cancers mostly arise in the reticulated epithelium-the specialized epithelium lining the tonsillar crypts. So, the HPV-related oropharyngeal cancers remain highly differentiated. The HPV negative HNSCC are of a heterogeneous group of benign and malignant lesions characterized by small tumour cells with round or ovoid nuclei surrounded by a thin rim of cytoplasm. On the other hand, HPV-related HNSCC encompasses basaloid cells. These cells exhibit lobular growth with dense hyperchromatic nuclei and a high nuclear to cytoplasmic ratio [15]. A recent study has shown that the "basaloid" subtype is, in fact, composed of a mixed group of HPV-positive and HPV-negative cancers that widely differ with respect to clinical behaviour [16].

2.1.2 Risk factors

Various epidemiological studies have revealed a diverse range of HNSCC associated risk factors. These risk factors include tobacco consumption, alcohol abuse, exposure to environmental pollutants and infection with viral agents namely, Human Papilloma Virus and Epstein Barr Virus (EBV). Certain risk factors show geographical, cultural and habitual prevalence [10]. Among the Asian population, oral cavity cancer is attributed to chewing of areca nut products including 'betel quid'-variety of customized mixtures comprising areca nut (Areca catechu, the carcinogen source), betel leaf (the leaf of Piper betel), slaked lime and/or tobacco, as well as spices according to local custom [17]. In common, the high male to female ratios for HPV-negative HNSCC incidence reflects the sex-specific patterns of variable risk behaviours, including the use of the aforesaid tobacco, smokeless tobacco, areca nut, betel quid and alcohol [17]. The additional risk factors that contribute to HNSCC include ageing, poor oral hygiene and diets lacking in vegetables [18]. In terms of the infectious agents that causes HNSCC, continuous infection with HPV and EBV can cause a rise in the cancers of Oropharynx and Nasopharynx [10]. The HPV infection that leads to HNSCC is mainly transmitted by oral sex and the occurrence of HPV-positive HNSCC continues to increase, especially in populations that are not vaccinated against HPV prior to HPV exposure [19]. Certain genetic factors have also been reviewed to contribute to HNSCC risk. Individuals with Fanconi anaemia, a rare, inherited genetic disease characterized by impaired DNA repair, have a 500- to 700-fold increased risk of developing HNSCC, primarily in the oral cavity [10].

2.1.3 Genetic differences

Frequent loss of chromosome arms 3p, 9p and amplification of 11q13 chromosomal region are observed in HNSCC. The key genes which are reported to be mutated by comprehensive genomic sequencing studies for Head and Neck squamous cell carcinoma are *TP53, PIK3CA, PTEN, FBXW7, HRAS*. The composition of chromosomal aberrations and mutations differs between HPV-positive and HPV-negative HNSCC. The *TP53* gene is the most frequently mutated gene (41%), and this gene was not detected in the HPV-positive subgroup. *PIK3CA* pathway is the frequently mutated oncogenic pathway in Head and Neck squamous cell carcinoma. Mutations in the *PIK3CA* pathway are slightly higher in the HPV-positive Head and squamous cell carcinoma. Mutations in *PIK3CA* and *PTEN* gene occur in both HPV-positive and HPV-negative patients but with slightly higher rates in HPV-positive patients [11]. Certain chromosomal aberrations include loss of 16q or 16q24.3, 5q35.1 or 17p12, 3q26.3. Loss of 9p21 containing the tumour suppressor gene *CDKN2A* is discerned in HPV negative HNSCC. The amplification of chromosome 7 is mutually exclusive for HPV-negative tumours [12]. CpG transversions are observed in HPV-negative HNSCC while TpC mutations are identified in HPV-positive HNSCC.

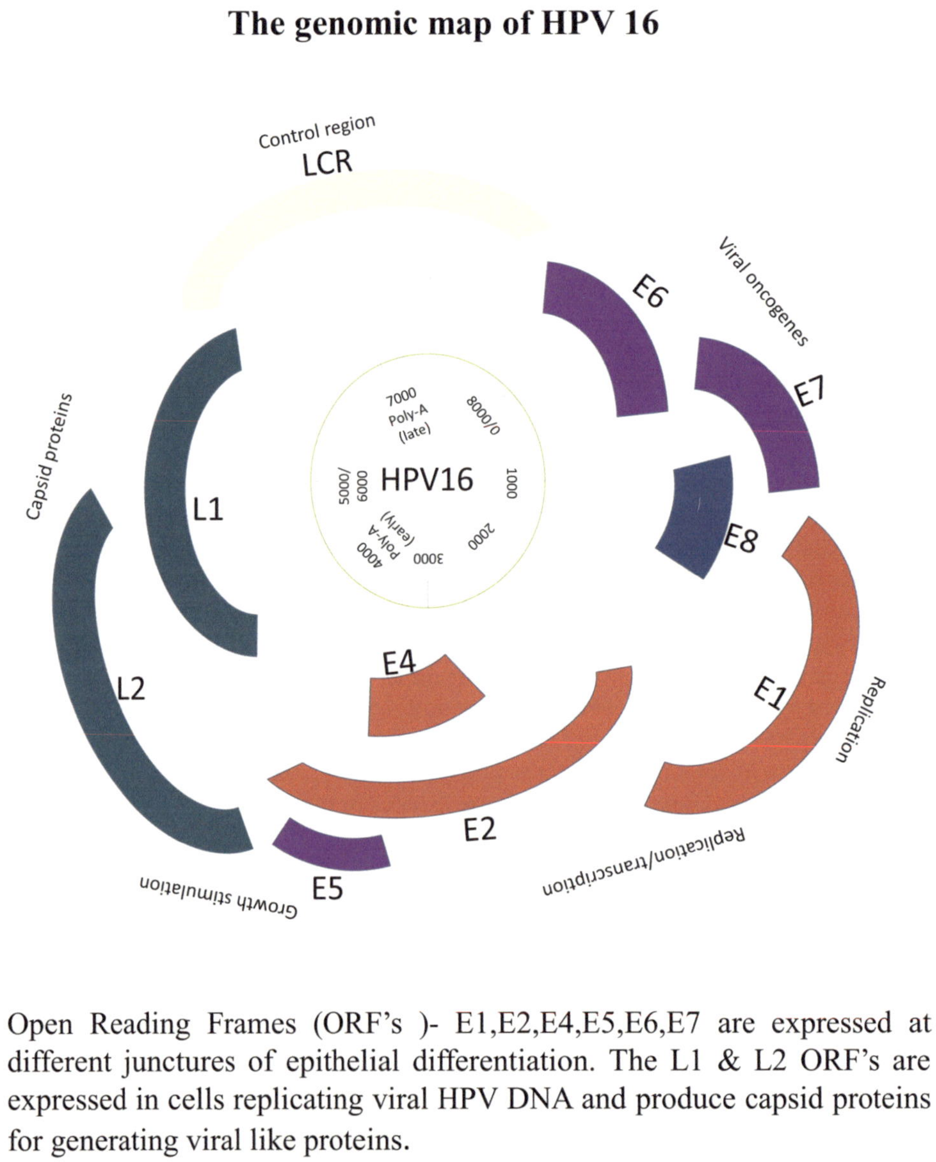

Figure 1.
The Genomic Map of HPV 16.

DOI: http://dx.doi.org/10.5772/intechopen.103737

HPV proteins	Functions
Early proteins	
E1	Initiation of viral genome replication.
E2	Viral DNA replication and transcription. Segregation of viral genomes.
E4	Viral genome packing. Maturation of viral particles.
E5	Oncoprotein. Participates in host cell transformation and blocks apoptosis in late events of HPV carcinogenesis.
E6	Major oncoprotein. Inactivates p53 protein. Block apoptosis. Interacts with many host proteins with PDZ domains.
E7	Major oncoprotein. Inactivates pRb protein. Promotes host DNA synthesis and proliferation. Interacts with many host proteins
Late proteins	
L1	Major capsid protein, Viral replicating proteins
L2	Minor capsid protein. Viral replicating proteins

Table 1.
HPV proteins and functions.

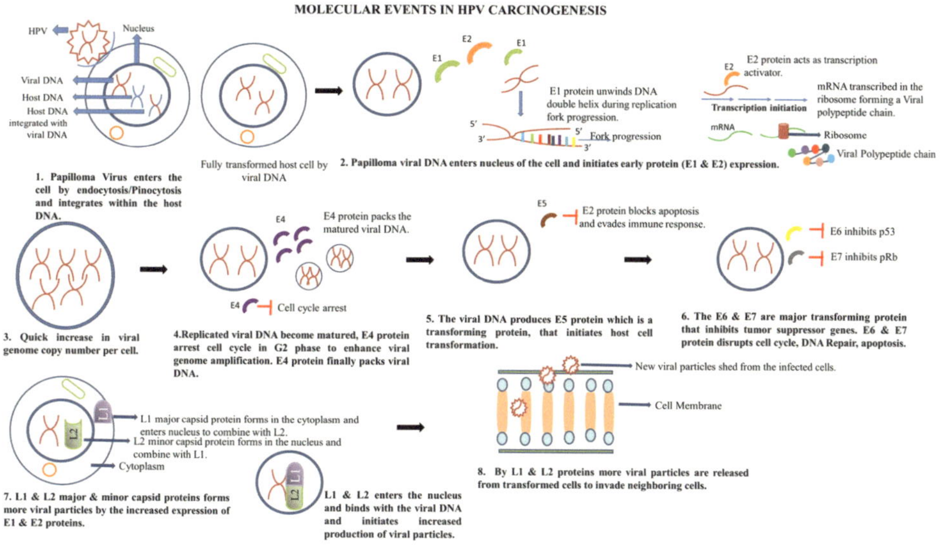

Figure 2.
Molecular events in HPV carcinogenesis.

2.1.4 Protein expression

The protein expression alterations in HPV- positive and HPV-negative groups showed a low expression of biomarker proteins such as MGMT, EGFR, and PD1-positive TILs in HPV positive and negative patients. Overexpression of EGFR protein is reported in HNSCC resulting in treatment resistance, aggressive clinical behaviour, and poor prognosis. The immunomodulatory protein PD-1 positivity occurs with highest frequency in pharyngeal cancers and PDL1 levels are detected in higher levels in nasopharyngeal cancers [11]. Patients with HPV positive tumours ensues abrogation of p53 and retinoblastoma (Rb) genes. The downregulation of the Rb gene results in the upregulation of p16 oncoprotein. The p16 oncoprotein is considered a biomarker for HPV-related HNSCC, where it is overexpressed. The minichromosomal maintenance protein 7 (MCM7) is expressed in high levels in HPV-positive head and neck cancer [19]. The p21 protein expression is identified in the HPV related tonsillar cancer. Reduced expression of p21 results in E6-mediated p53 inactivation. Outcomes from other studies indicate that E7 bypasses the inhibitory effect of p21 on cell cycle progression [20, 21]. Survivin (Baculoviral IAP repeat-containing protein 5) is negatively regulated by p53. This protein represses apoptosis and plays a role in cell division. Nuclear survivin expression is associated with a poor disease-free survival

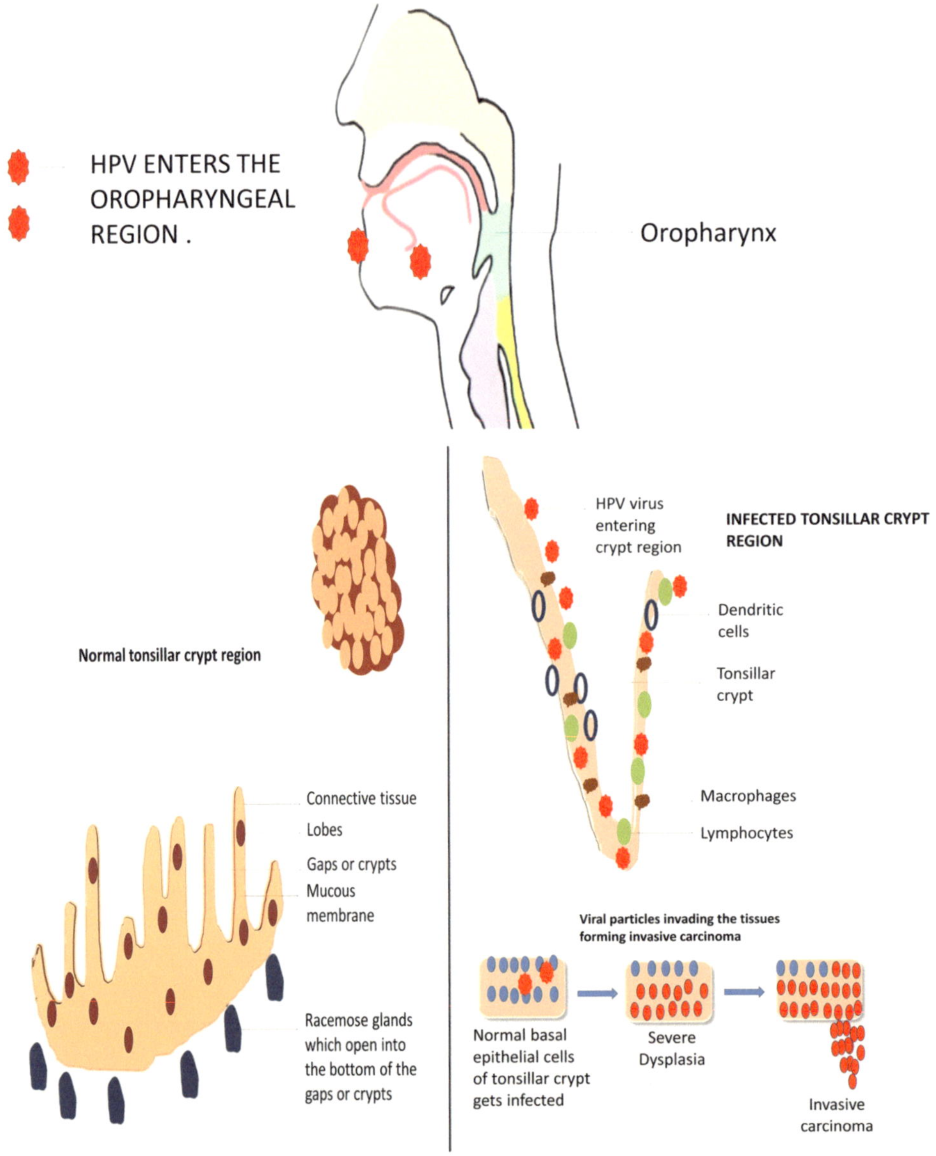

Figure 3.
HPV transformation via Tonsillar crypt.

rate and negative HPV status in OPSCC [22]. Thioredoxin (TRX) (redox mediator promoting cell survival) and epidermal fatty acid binding protein (E-FABP) involved in keratinocyte differentiation and other cellular signaling processes were perceived to be upregulated in HPV-related tumours and their role in HPV-related OSCC. Several cell surface glycoprotein molecular biomarkers such as CD44, CD133, ALDH1 occurs in elevated level in HNSCC. The HNSCC cells with high levels of CD44 glycoproteins are capable of self-renewal. CD44 levels in HNSCC tumours are associated with metastasis and a poor prognosis [23, 24]. CD133 glycoproteins results in increased invasiveness and metastasis in HNSCC. The increased levels of ALDH1 causes self-renewal, invasiveness and metastasis in HNSCC (**Figures 1–3** and **Table 1**) [25].

2.2 Mutational profile of head and neck squamous cell carcinoma (HNSCC)

2.2.1 Common genetic alterations in HNSCC

The common cytogenetic changes observed in head and neck cancers are losses of segments of 3p, 5q, 8p, 9p, 10p, and 18q and gains of segments within 3q, 5p, 7p, 8q, distal 1q, and 11q13–23 regions.

Amplifications of 11q13 and 7p11 regions encoding *Cyclin D1* and *EGFR* respectively are noted in HNSCC [26]. Telomerase Reverse Transcriptase (*TERT*) found on chromosome 5p and *MYC* oncogene on 8q region of the chromosome exhibits additional amplification in both HPV positive and HPV negative HNSCC [27]. Portions of chromosomes 3P and 8P which encompasses the tumour suppressor genes *FHIT* and *CSMD1* respectively are deleted in HNSCC [28].

The microRNA let-7c, a cell cycle regulator, is frequently inactivated in both HPV negative and HPV positive HNSCC. Decreased expression of let7-c is linked with increased expression of CDK4, CDK6, E2F1 and PLK1 kinases and translational regulators important for advancement through the cell cycle [29].

2.2.2 Genetic alterations in HPV associated HNSCC

Molecular heterogeneity has been found to exist within HPV (+) tumours themselves. High rate of proliferation and increase in genomic instability is associated with HPV integration [30]. Human papilloma virus induced tumourigenesis occurs predominantly in the oropharynx region (tonsil or base of tongue), where HPV acquired oncoproteins E6 and E7 inactivate the tumour suppressor genes *p53* and *pRb* (retinoblastoma), resulting in the inception and eventual progression to malignancy [31].

HPV positive HNSCC are characterized by wild-type TP53. High-risk types HPV encode two viral oncoproteins namely E6 and E7 that aid tumour progression by inactivating the two well-characterized tumour suppressor proteins TP53 and RB1, respectively. Un-phosphorylated RB1 plays a crucial role in the negative regulation of cell proliferation, generating cell cycle arrest in mid to late G_1. Wild-type TP53 behaves as a cell cycle checkpoint after DNA damage and induces G_1 arrest or apoptosis, essential to conserve the genomic stability [32]. However, HPV-associated cancers normally do not manifest *TP53* mutations.

PIK3CA (protein kinase C), an anti-apoptotic kinase and transcription factors *TP63* and *SOX2* located on chromosome 3q are among the most frequently amplified regions in HPV associated Head and Neck Squamous Cell Carcinoma(HNSCC) [33]. *PIK3CA* encodes the p110α catalytic subunit of phosphinositol-3-kinase. Regulation of signal from multiple input sources including many of the receptor tyrosine kinases (RTKs) relevant to HNSCC is advocated by *PIK3CA* through phosphorylation of AKT1. Mutated *PIK3CA* has been shown to impair apoptotic signals and support tumour invasion. Additionally, mutational turned on *PIK3CA* has been shown to assist cyclin D activity, further emphasizing cell cycle deregulation in head and neck cancers [34].

Meagre or no *EGFR* gene amplification and *EGFR* protein expression has been observed in HPV-positive HNSCC [35]. HPV (+) tumours manifest infrequent mutations in *TP53* gene.

Truncating mutations are observed in TNF receptor-associated factor 3 (*TRAF3*) gene which is implicated in anti-viral responses (innate and acquired) of Human Papilloma Virus (HPV) [36]. *TRAF3* region is absolutely lost in about 20% of HPV-associated tumours. Tumour necrosis factor Receptor-Associated Factor 3 (*TRAF3*, encoded on 14q32.32) is involved in the innate and acquired antiviral immune response in HPV positive HNSCC. Deletion or mutations in *TRAF3* genes is over-represented in HPV-related HNSCC. As genes coding for HLA I components are frequently mutated and higher numbers of CD56-positive natural killer cells have been reported for HPV-related Oropharyngeal Squamous Cell Carcinoma recently innate immunity seems to be eloquent for HPV-related HNSCC [37].

Amplification of E2F1 region which is necessary for cell cycle initiation and proliferation and an intact 9p21.3 region containing the CDKN2A gene are observed in the HPV positive HNSCC [38].

TpC mutations were observed predominantly in HPV associated HNSCC patients during the whole exome sequence analysis. These TpC mutations lead to APOBEC mutational signature in HPV positive HNSCC [38]. Overexpression of APOBEC enzymes in HPV-associated tumours may be linked to increased cytosine deaminase mutation [39]. Genes encoding HLA I components are frequently mutated in HPV positive Oropharyngeal Squamous Cell Carcinoma (OPSCC) [39]. Sewell et al. [40] in 2014 screened eleven DNA repair proteins which included *BRCA2*, *PARP-1*, and *MSH2 ATM* and observed all of them to be upregulated in HPV positive OPSCC samples compared to the HPV negative OPSCC samples.

2.2.3 Inactivating mutations in HPV-positive HNSCC

Segregation of four genes are observed as inactivating mutations in HPV positive tumours of which two genes *CDKN2A* and *TP53* are associated with survival and cell cycle and two genes *FAT1* and *AJUBA* with Wnt/b-catenin signalling [41]. A higher rate of TP53 mutations are observed in HPV positive HNSCC compared to non-HPV associated HNSCC.

2.2.4 Genetic alterations in non-HPV associated HNSCC

HPV negative HNSCC tumours features novel co-amplifications of 11q13 (*CCND1*, *FADD* and *CTTN*) and 11q22 (*BIRC2* and *YAP1*), which also contain genes implicated in cell death/NF-κB and Hippo pathways. They also emphasize novel focal deletions in the nuclear set domain gene (*NSD1*) and tumour suppressor genes like *FAT1*, *NOTCH1*, *SMAD4* and *CDKN2A*. Recurrent focal amplifications in receptor tyrosine kinases like *EGFR*, *ERBB2* and *FGFR1* also predominate in HPV negative HNSCC tumours [38].

Cyclin-dependent kinase inhibitor 2A (also known as p16 INK4A) that is encoded by *CDKN2A* gene located at 9p21, is frequently inactivated *via* copy number loss among HPV-negative head and neck cancer patients and is involved in the HNSCC pathogenesis. *CDKN2A* regulates cell cycle progression by obstructing the activity of *CCND1* (cyclin D1) and its related kinases, CDK6 and CDK4. These kinases are involved in the phosphorylation and inactivation of the tumour suppressor gene *RB1* *CDKN2A* hinders cell cycle progression at the G1 to S check point by preventing the phosphorylation of the retinoblastoma protein (*RB1*). Deletion, mutation or hyper-methylation of *CDKN2A* is frequent in HPV negative HNSCC and is associated with worse prognosis in these Head and Neck cancers [34]. On the other hand, *CDKN2A* overexpression has been correlated with improved outcome in Oropharyngeal Squamous Cell Carcinoma. This occurs as an outcome of functional inactivation of *RB1* by the HPV E7 protein, resulting in the upregulation of *CDKN2A* [42]. Thus, HPV positive HNSCC are characterized by high expression of *CDKN2A*, implying that *CDKN2A* positivity may be a biomarker for tumours harboring HPV infections [42]. Inactivation of the *CDKN2A* gene has been found in 57% of HPV negative HNSCC cases in the TCGA cohort [38].

The transmembrane receptor protein *NOTCH1* is involved in cell proliferation, differentiation, cell fate determination and self-destruction Additionally, Notch plays a decisive role in angiogenesis, crucial for the maintenance and progression of tumourigenesis. NOTCH1 inactivation has been inferred in about 15% of the HNSCC tumours. Most NOTCH1 mutations in HNSCC are considered inactivating, attributing its role as a tumour suppressor gene. On the contrary, cohorts from Asian HNSCC population have demonstrated activating NOTCH1 mutations. NOTCH activity in HNSCC is therefore circumstantial and NOTCH is considered to have a bimodal role as a tumour suppressor and an oncogene in HNSCC. HNSCC with NOTCH1 mutations have a worse prognosis than the NOTCH1 wild-type tumours. Most studies reveal that *NOTCH* pathway is upregulated in HNSCC and *NOTCH* expression shows convincing relationship with the clinical stage [43]. The *NOTCH* pathway can play an influential role in HNSCC development, and anti-*NOTCH* therapy can be attractive. *NOTCH1* is observed to be more mutated in HPV-negative HNSCC than in HPV-positive HNSCC [44]. Higher expression of *NOTCH1* is displayed in HPV-positive HNSCC compared to HPV-negative HNSCC.

The region of epidermal growth factor receptor (*EGFR*) gene is 7p12 and it encodes for a 170-kD transmembrane glycoprotein. It is a member of the receptor protein tyrosine kinase family with several extracellular growth factor ligands, comprising of epidermal growth factor (EGF) and transforming growth factor (TGF)-α. About 42–80% of HNSCC studied has overexpression of EGFR [26], and 30% of HNSCC tumours *have been discerned to harbor EGFR* gene amplification. Increased EGFR expression and gene copy number are associated with poorer patient outcomes in HNSCC.

Mutations in genes *NFE2L2* (encoding NRF2) and *KEAP1* occur exclusively in HPV-negative HNSCC. These two genes are known key regulators of oxidative stress. CpG transversions are frequent in HPV-negative HNSCC.

H-RAS mutation is detected in about 35% of Indian oral cancer patients. This gene has been associated with betel nut chewing and so observed in HPV-negative HNSCC. Also, somatic mutation at codon 12 of *K-ras* gene makes the *K-ras* protein hyper active, leading to uncontrolled signalling for cell division (**Tables 2** and **3**) [45].

2.3 Epigenetic alterations in HPV-positive and HPV-negative HNSCC

Epigenetic events of HNSCC include DNA methylation, chromatin remodelling, histone posttranslational covalent modifications and effects of non-coding RNA.

Epigenetics sway silencing of tumour suppressor genes by promoter hypermethylation, regulate transcription by microRNAs and changes in chromatin structure, or induce genome instability through hypomethylation. Most of the HNSCC are caused by hypomethylation of the promoter genes or retrotransposons. Lower methylation of retrotransposons elements such as LINE (long interspersed elements) and SINE (short interspersed elements) causes the initiation of tumour in HNSCC. It is also reported that hypomethylation is concerned with tongue squamous cell carcinoma (TSCC) among the female gender [51]. The hypomethylation of Alu, one of the SINEs, is reported in the oral cancer patients of Asian population in the advanced stages of cancer [52]. Further, patients with severe malignant oral carcinogenesis are associated with hypomethylation of LINE sequences [53]. The hypermethylation in HNSCC implicate a high level of methylation in promoters of genes, which is a characteristic feature for epigenomes of cancer cells. Hypermethylation of certain genes

TCGA [38]		**Seiwert et al. [46]**		**Stransky et al. [47]**		**Agrawal et al. [43]**
HPV (+ve)	**HPV (−ve)**	**HPV (+ve)**	**HPV (−ve)**	**HPV (+ve)**	**HPV (−ve)**	**HPV (+ve)**
E6/E7 (100%)	TP53 (84%, M)	E6/E7 (100%)	TP53 (81%, M)	E6/E7 (100%)	TP53 (73%, M)	E6/E7 (100%)
PIK3CA (56%, M/A)	CDKN2A (57%, M/D)	PIK3CA (22%, M)	CDKN2A (33%, M/D)	PIK3CA (27%, M)	CDKN2A (25%, M/D)	EPHB3 (25%, M)
TP63 (28%, A)	let-7c (40%, miRNA)	TP63 (16%, M/A)	MDM2 (16%, A)	RUFY1 (18%, M)	SYNE1 (22%, M)	UNC5D (25%, M)
TRAF3 (22%, M/D)	PIK3CA (34%, M/A)	PIK3CB (13%, M/A)	MLL2 (16%, M)	EZH2 (18%, M)	CCND1 (22%, A)	NLRP12 (25%, M)
E2F1 (19%, A)	FADD (32%, A)	FGFR3 (14%, M)	NOTCH 1 (16%, M)	CDH10 (18%, M)	MUC16 (19%, M)	PIK3CA (25%, M)
let-7c (17%, miRNA)	FAT1 (32%, M/D)	NF1/2 (12%, M)	CCND1 (13%, A)	THSD7A (18%, M)	USH2A (18%, M)	TM7SF3 (25%, M)
NOTCH1/3 (17%, M)	CCND1 (31%, A)	SOX2 (12%, A)	PIK3CA (13%, M)	FAT4 (18%, M)	FAT1 (14%, M)	ENPP1 (25%, M)
FGFR3 (11%, F/M)	NOTCH1/2/3 (29%, M/D)	ATM (10%, D)	PIK3CB (13%, M/A)	KMT2D (18%, M)	LRP1B (14%, M)	NRXN3 (25%, M)
HLA-A/B (11%, M/D)	TP63 (19%, A)	FLG (12%, M)	UBR5 (13%, M/D)	ZNF676 (18%, M)	ZFHX4 (14%, M)	MICAL2 (25%, M)
EGFR (6%, M)	EGFR (15%, M/A)	MLL3 (10%, M)	EGFR (12%, A)	MUC16 (18%, M)	NOTCH1 (13%, M)	—

M, mutation; A, amplification; D, deletion; F, fusion.

Table 2.
Genes altered in HPV-positive and HPV-negative HNSCC.

Lin et al. [48]	Pickering et al. [49]		Pickering et al. [50]
Nasopharyngeal cancer (NPC)	Tongue		Oral squamous cell carcinoma (OSCC)
	Young tongue	Old tongue	
CDKN2A/B (13%, M/D)	TP53 (94%, M)	TP53 (57%, M)	CDKN2A (74%, D)
ARID1A (11%, M/D)	CSMD1 (25%,D)	CSMD1 (75%,D	TP53 (66%, M)
SYNE1 (8%, M)	PIK3CA (0%, M); (30%A)	PIK3CA (11%, M); (70%, A)	FAT1 (46%, M/D)
ATG13 (6%, M/D)	CDKN2A (6%, M); (55%, D)	CDKN2A (4%, M); (65%, D)	TP63 (26%, A)
MLL2 (6%, M)	FADD/CCND1 (40%, A)	FADD/CCND1 (65%, A)	CCND1 (23%, A)
PIK3CA (6%, M/A)	FAT1 (6%, M); (50%, D)	FAT1 (25%, M); (35%, D)	MAML1 (23%, D)
CCND1 (4%, A)	EGFR (20%, A)	EGFR (50%, A)	EGFR (17%, A)
NOTCH3 (4%, M)	NOTCH1 (25%, M)	NOTCH1 (18%, M)	TNK2 (17%, A)
FGFR2 (4%, M)	HLA-A (0%, M)	HLA-A (14%, M)	AKT1 (14%, A)
TP53 (17%, M/D)	CASP8 (6%, M)	CASP8 (11%, M)	SRC (14%, A)

M, mutation; A, amplification; D, deletion; F, fusion.

Table 3.
Altered genes in different anatomic sites of HNSCC irrespective of HPV infection.

such as *CDKN2A*, *PTEN, DAPK, MGMT, ECAD* and *RASSF1* are frequently observed in HNSCC [54]. This increased methylation is associated with well-differentiated tumours and with patient age less than 50 years in OSCC among Indian population [55]. There occurs difference in methylation status among HPV-positive and HPV-negative patients. Studies have reported that HPV infection causes aberrant hyper or hypo methylation of genes. The study reports obtained from genome-wide methylation data from different cohorts showed that HPV infection affects DNA methylation in HNSCC across different anatomic sites. Only a few hypomethylated genes have been reported in HNSCC cases that are HPV infected. Two miRNAs, miR-875 and miR-3144 found in E6 gene, inhibit E6 oncogene expression, and in HPV16-positive cell lines inhibit the growth and promote apoptosis by high-level expression of both miRNAs (**Table 4**) [56].

3. Pathways involved in HNSCC

3.1 EGFR pathway

In HNSCC, activation of EGFR is executed by binding of ligands such as EGF, amphiregulin, and transforming growth factor alpha-TGFα. Ligand binding provokes receptor dimerization (homo or hetero dimerization with other EGFR members), leading to phosphorylation of tyrosine residues. This leads to sequential activation of various signalling cascades like Ras/Raf/mitogen-activated protein kinase (MAPK), phosphoinositide 3-kinase (PI3K)-Akt, signal transducer and activator of transcription pathways. Phosphorylated MAPK translocates into the nucleus, phosphorylating various transcription factors that

Mirghani et al. [60]	Hui et al. [61]	Gao et al. [62]	Lajer et al. [63]	Gao et al. [64]
miR-324-5p	miR-324-5p		miR-324-5p	
	miR-155	miR-155	miR-155	
miR-107	miR-107			
	miR-9	miR-9		
	miR-145			miR-145
miR-99b-3p			miR-99b-3p	
miR-18a-5p		miR-18a-5p		
			miR-26b	miR-26b
			miR-363	miR-363
	miR-381			miR-381
	miR-101			miR-101

Table 4.
Deregulated miRNAs in HNSCC irrespective of HPV infection.

trigger the expression of distinct target genes, which advocates proliferation, differentiation, migration, invasion, angiogenesis and metastasis in HNSCC cells. Aberration of EGFR signal activation can bring about disruption of cancer cell homeostasis [57–59].

3.2 PI3K-AKT mTOR pathway

Activated by the receptor-associated tyrosine kinases (RTKs) such as EGFR, the catalytic subunit phosphorylates phosphatidylinositol 1, 4-bisphosphate (PIP2) to phosphatidylinositol 1, 4, 5-triphosphate (PIP3). PIP3 recruits proteins like phosphoinositide-dependent protein kinase 1 (PDK1) and AKT to the plasma membrane, resulting in the phosphorylation of AKT by PDK1 and mammalian target of rapamycin complex 2 (mTORC2). Activated AKT and mTORC1 in turn activates the eukaryotic translation inhibition factor 4E-binding protein 1 (4E-BP1), resulting in cell growth, protein synthesis, and proliferation of HNSCC. The tumour suppressor phosphatase and tensin homology (PTEN) negatively regulates the cellular level of PIP3 by converting it to PIP2 through its lipid phosphatase activity thereby negating the activation of AKT and its downstream pathways. More than 80% of mutations occur in exon 9 (Helical domain) and exon 20 (Kinase domain) through gene amplification mechanism and increase in low-level copy number. More invasive forms of HNSCC have been proclaimed to harbour copy number increase in 3q26 region and engage in vascular invasion and lymph node metastasis. Oncogenic PIK3CA mutations are common particularly in HPV-positive head and neck cancers. PIK3CA mutations may combine with E6 and E7 proteins of HPV in the evolution of invasive OPSCC [57–59].

3.3 p53/Rb/CDKN2A/CCND1 pathway

In HNSCC, TP53 has been linked with the risk of progression from mild dysplasia to invasive carcinoma. P53 level is determined by MDM2, which by ubiquitination degrades p53. Contrarily, p14 and p16 encoded by CDKN2A inhibits MDM2 and

DOI: http://dx.doi.org/10.5772/intechopen.103737

shields p53 from degradation. RB inhibits E2F transcription factor from progressing into the cell cycle. Cyclin and cyclin-dependent kinases (CDK) like D1/CDK4/CDK6 are activated by mitotic signals which leads to the inactivation of RB via phosphorylation. p21 (CDKN1) and p16 (INK4A/MTS1/CDKN2) encoded by CDKN2A inhibits Cyclin D1-CDK4/6 complex. Phosphorylation of RB results in release of E2F and cell cycle progresses to S, G2 and M phases. Inactivation of p53, RB, p16 and p14 through mutation, deletion or epigenetic silencing and overexpression of cyclin D1 (CCND1 gene), MDM2 and CDK4 have been associated with tumorigenesis and reduced survival in HNSCC. HPV infection can inhibit the activation of p53 and RB in HNSCC. Seven early proteins (E1–E7) and two late capsid proteins (L1 and L2) are encoded by HPV genome.

HPV E6 combines with E6-associated protein (E6-AP) and endorses p53 ubiquitin proteasome degradation. For binding to RB, HPV E7 protein encounters with E2F. As RB acts as a negative regulator for the cyclin-dependent kinase inhibitor p16, overexpression of p16 has been established to be of great clinical value in determining the HPV-positive status of the tumours using immunohistochemistry (IHC) (**Figure 4**) [57–59].

3.4 NOTCH pathway

The NOTCH family consists of four receptors (NOTCH1-4) adhered to the cell membrane. They are activated by two families of ligands, namely, Delta-like (Dll1, DllL3, Dll4) and Jagged (Jag1 and Jag2). Binding of ligands to NOTCH receptors persuade NOTCH cleavage by TNFα-converting enzyme (TACE) (ADAM metalloprotease) and γ-secretase, which results in the release of NOTCH intracellular domain (NICD). NICD associates with CSL/MAM complex, binds to DNA and promotes transcription. NOTCH pathway is a conserved signal transduction cascade which alters cell function such as cell differentiation, survival and self-renewal capacity. Notch activity has been associated with the suppression of HPV E6 and E7 protein expression, leading to for

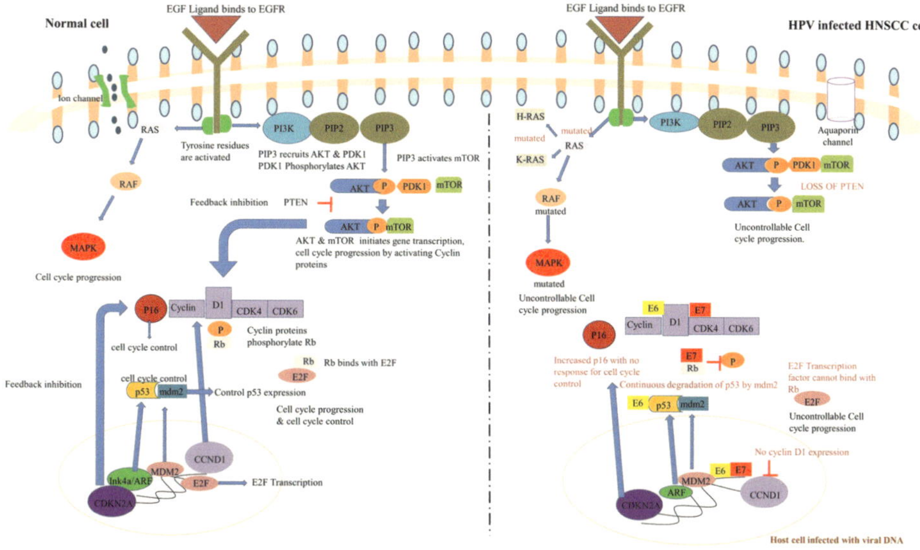

Figure 4.
EGFR, PI3K-AKT- mTOR, p53/Rb/CDKN2A/CCND1 pathways.

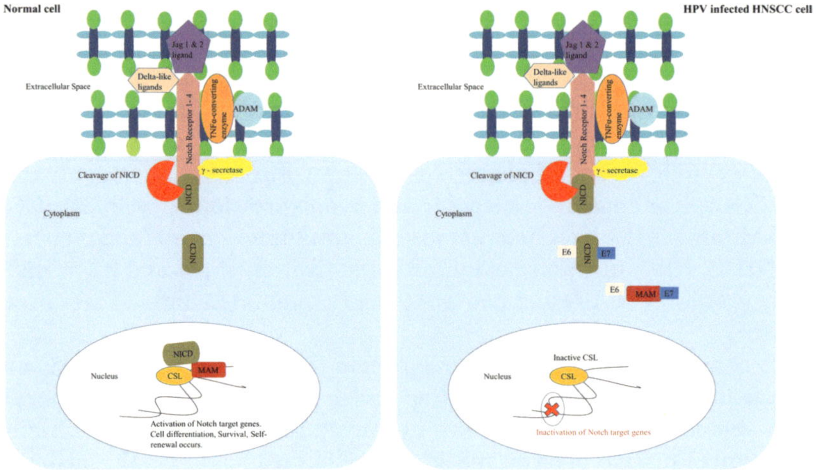

Figure 5.
NOTCH pathway.

loss of Notch in HPV+ HNSCC. NOTCH1 signalling stimulates terminal differentiation of keratinocytes and it is negatively regulated by EGFR pathway (**Figure 5**) [57–59].

4. Conclusion

Based upon the research studies till date there is a clear evidence portraying that the high risk HPV types are well known for causing Head and neck squamous cell carcinoma. The studies have also proved the HPV Viral infection within the different anatomic sites; among the different anatomic sites the oropharyngeal region has a major impact of getting huge amount of viral load thus causing HPV infection. The infected virus further initiates transformation process within the oropharyngeal region such as the oropharynx (51%), pharynx (5%), and oral cavity (9%). The viral makeover within the oral cavity occurs in the tonsillar crypt epithelium and integrates within the human genome. Estimates have shown that there accounts huge amount of HPV viral-cellular entry within the tonsillar crypt epithelium. Several studies have revealed that there occurs physiological differences between HPV-positive and HPV-negative HNSCC, thus differing with respect to clinical behaviour. Certain risk factors influence HPV-positive and HPV-negative HNSCC. The HPV-negative oral cavity cancer is attributed to chewing of areca nut products, betel leaf (the leaf of Piper betel), slaked lime and/or tobacco. Smoking is also contributed to causing HPV-negative HNSCC. The HPV-positive risk factors include continuous infection with HPV and EBV which usually arise in the cancers of Oropharynx and Nasopharynx. HPV infections occur in higher rate mainly due to oral sex, and people who have not been vaccinated. Research findings have revealed that there occurs difference in genes being mutated in HPV-positive and HPV-negative HNSCC. The most common genes mutated within HPV-positive and HPV-negative HNSCC include *TP53*, *PIK3CA*, *PTEN*, *FBXW7*, *HRAS*. Among these the *TP53* has the highest mutations in HPV-negative HNSCC and in HPV-positive HNSCC the E6/E7 viral proteins has the highest integration in the human genome, the *PIK3CA* gene has a profound mutation levels in HPV-positive HNSCC. Studies on the epigenetic alterations in HPV-positive and HPV-negative HNSCC reveal differentially expressed miRNAs. The methylation characteristics of HNSCC illustrate a variation in hypermethylation and hypomethylation levels in HPV-positive and HPV-negative HNSCC. Further the methylation status differs among the anatomic sites of HNSCC. The integration of HPV within human genome causes an aberrant expression of proteins among the different anatomic sites. It has been reported that the viral proteins E6 suppresses p53 gene and E7 suppresses Rb gene. These two genes are involved in several normal regulatory cell cycles. Patients with HPV positive and Tobacco-associated HNSCC ensues abrogation of p53 and retinoblastoma (Rb) genes. There occurs other immunomodulatory proteins elevated in HPV-negative HNSCC and in HPV-positive HNSCC, PD-1 and PDL1 detected in higher levels in nasopharyngeal cancers, pharyngeal cancers. Thus the studies on the HPV-positive and HPV-negative HNSCC with regard to their anatomical, physiological, genetic, proteomic characteristics can bring out novel treatment strategies. Further molecular and genetic studies are required to bring out unknown facts within the HPV-positive and HPV-negative HNSCC. The so far obtained data can be implemented in future diagnostic and clinical applications.

Abbreviations

ADAM	a disintegrin and metalloproteinases
AJUBA	Ajuba LIM Protein
AKT1	v-akt murine thymoma viral oncogenes homolg 1
ALDH1	aldehyde dehydrogenase 1
APOBEC	apolipoprotein B mRNA-editing enzyme catalytic polypeptide
ARID1A	AT-rich interaction domain 1A
ATG13	autophagy-related protein 13
ATM	ataxia telangiectasia mutated
BIRC2	baculoviral IAP repeat containing 2
BRCA2	BReast CAncer gene 2
CASP8	cysteine-aspartic acid protease (caspase) family
CCND1	cyclin D1
CD133	cluster of differentiation 133
CD44	cluster of differentiation 44
CD56	cluster of differentiation 56
CDH10	Cadherin 10
CDK4	cyclin-dependent kinase 4
CDK6	cell division protein kinase 6
CDKN2A	cyclin-dependent kinase inhibitor 2A
CSMD1	CUB and Sushi multiple domains 1
CTTN	cortactin
DAPK	death-associated protein kinase 1
E2F1	E2F transcription factor 1
ECAD	epithelial cadherin (E-cadherin)
E-FABP	epidermal fatty acid binding protein
EGFR	epidermal growth factor receptor
ENPP1	ectonucleotide pyrophosphatase/phosphodiesterase 1
EPHB3	ephrin type-B receptor 3
ERBB2	receptor tyrosine-protein kinase erbB-2
EZH2	enhancer of Zeste 2 polycomb repressive complex 2 subunit

FADD	Fas associated via death domain
FAT1	FAT atypical cadherin 1
FBXW7	F-box and wd repeat domain containing 7
FGFR1	fibroblast growth factor receptor 1
FGFR3	fibroblast growth factor receptor 3
FHIT	fragile histidine triad
FLG	filaggrin
HLA I	human leukocyte antigen
HNSCC	Head and Neck Squamous Cell Carcinoma
HPV	Human Papillomavirus
HRAS	Harvey rat sarcoma viral oncogenes homolog
KEAP1	Kelch-like ECH-associated protein 1
KMT2D	lysine methyltransferase 2D
LINE	long interspersed elements
LRP1B	low-density lipoprotein receptor-related protein 1B
MCM7	minichromosomal maintenance protein 7
MDM2	mouse double minute 2 homolog
MGMT	O6-methylguanine DNA methyltransferase
MICAL2	Microtubule Associated Monooxygenase Calponin and LIM Domain Containing 2
MLL2	histone-lysine N-methyltransferase MLL2
MSH2	MutS homolog 2
MUC16	Mucin 16 cell surface associated
MYC	MYC proto-oncogene
NF1/2	neurofibromatosis type 1
NFE2L2	nuclear factor erythroid 2-related factor 2
NICD	NOTCH intracellular domain
NLRP12	NLR Family Pyrin Domain Containing 12
NOTCH1	Notch homolog 1 translocation-associated (Drosophila)
NRF2	nuclear factor erythroid 2-related factor 2
NRXN3	Neurexin 3
NSD1	nuclear receptor binding SET domain protein 1
OPSCC	Oropharyngeal Squamous Cell Carcinoma
PARP-1	poly [ADP-ribose] polymerase 1
PCR	Polymerase Chain Reaction
PD1	PDCD1; programmed cell death 1
PDL1	programmed cell death ligand 1
PI3KCA	phosphatidylinositol-45-bisphosphate 3-kinase catalytic subunit alpha
PIK3CB	phosphatidylinositol-4,5-Bisphosphate 3-Kinase Catalytic Subunit Beta
PISH	PCR *in situ* hybridization
PTEN	phosphatase and tensin homolog
RASSF1	Ras Association Domain Family Member 1
Rb	retinoblastoma
RTKs	receptor tyrosine kinases
RUFY1	RUN and FYVE domain containing 1
SINE	short interspersed elements
SMAD4	SMAD family member 4 mothers against decapentaplegic homolog 4
SOX2	sex determining region Y

SRC	proto-oncogene tyrosine-protein kinase sarcoma
SYNE1	spectrin repeat containing nuclear envelope protein 1
TERT	telomerase reverse transcriptase
THSD7A	thrombospondin type 1 domain containing 7A
TILs	Tumour infiltrating lymphocytes
TM7SF3	transmembrane 7 superfamily member 3
TNK2	tyrosine kinase non receptor 2
TP53	tumour protein p53
TRAF3	TNF receptor associated factor 3
TRX	thioredoxin
TSCC	tongue squamous cell carcinoma
UBR5	ubiquitin protein ligase E3 component N-recognin 5
UNC5D	Unc-5 netrin receptor D
USH2A	Usher syndrome type 2A
YAP1	yes-associated protein 1
ZFHX4	Zinc Finger Homeobox 4
ZNF676	zinc finger protein 676

Author details

Minu Jenifer Michael Raj, Fenwick Antony Edwin Rodrigues
and Sivasamy Ramasamy*
Department of Human Genetics and Molecular Biology, Bharathiar University,
Coimbatore Tamil Nadu, India

*Address all correspondence to: rshgmb@buc.edu.in

References

[1] Ferlay J, Colombet M, Soerjomataram I, Mathers C, Parkin DM, Piñeros M, et al. Estimating the global cancer incidence and mortality in 2018: GLOBOCAN sources and methods. International Journal of Cancer. 2019;**144**(8):1941-1953. DOI: 10.1002/ijc.31937

[2] Lacko M, Braakhuis BJM, Sturgis EM, Boedeker CC, Suárez C, Rinaldo A, et al. Genetic susceptibility to head and neck squamous cell carcinoma. International Journal of Radiation Oncology*Biology*Physics. 2014;**89**(1):38-48

[3] Michaud DS, Langevin SM, Eliot M, Nelson HH, Pawlita M, McClean MD, et al. High-risk HPV types and head and neck cancer. International Journal of Cancer. 2014;**135**(7):1653-1661. DOI: 10.1002/ijc

[4] Kobayashi K, Hisamatsu K, Suzui N, Hara A, Tomita H, Miyazaki T. A review of HPV-related head and neck cancer. Journal of Clinical Medicine. 2018;7(9):241. DOI: 10.3390/jcm7090241

[5] Wilczynski SP, Lin BT, Xie Y, Paz IB. Detection of human papillomavirus DNA and oncoprotein overexpression are associated with distinct morphological patterns of tonsillar squamous cell carcinoma. The American Journal of Pathology. 1998;**152**(1):145-156

[6] Gillison ML, Koch WM, Capone RB, Spafford M, Westra WH, Wu L, et al. Evidence for a causal association between human papillomavirus and a subset of head and neck cancers. Journal of the National Cancer Institute. 2000;**92**(9):709-720

[7] Braakhuis BJ, Snijders PJ, Keune WJ, Meijer CJ, Ruijter-Schippers HJ, Leemans CR, et al. Genetic patterns in head and neck cancers that contain or lack transcriptionally active human papillomavirus. Journal of the National Cancer Institute. 2004;**96**(13):998-1006

[8] Venuti A, Paolini F. HPV detection methods in head and neck cancer. Head and Neck Pathology. 2012;**Suppl. 1**:S63-S74. DOI: 10.1007/s12105-012-0372-5

[9] Huang SH, O'Sullivan B, Xu W, Zhao H, Chen DD, Ringash J, et al. Temporal nodal regression and regional control after primary radiation therapy for N2-N3 head-and-neck cancer stratified by HPV status. International Journal of Radiation Oncology, Biology, Physics. 2013;**87**(5):1078-1085. DOI: 10.1016/j.ijrobp.2013.08.049

[10] Johnson DE, Burtness B, Leemans CR, Lui VWY, Bauman JE, Grandis JR. Head and neck squamous cell carcinoma. Nature Reviews. Disease Primers. 2020;**6**(1):92. DOI: 10.1038/s41572-020-00224-3

[11] Feldman R, Gatalica Z, Knezetic J, Reddy S, Nathan C-A, Javadi N, et al. Molecular profiling of head and neck squamous cell carcinoma. Head & Neck. 2016;**38**:E1625-E1638. DOI: 10.1002/hed.24290

[12] Gillison M, D'Souza G, Westra W. Distinct risk factor profiles for human papillomavirus type 16–positive and human papillomavirus type 16–negative head and neck cancers. Journal of the National Cancer Institute. 2008;**100**:407-420

[13] Smith EM, Ritchie JM, Summersgill KF. Human papillomavirus in oral exfoliated cells and risk of head

and neck cancer. Journal of the National Cancer Institute. 2004;**96**:449-455

[14] Herrero R, Castellsague X, Pawlita M. Human papillomavirus and oral cancer: The international agency for research on cancer multicenter study. Journal of the National Cancer Institute. 2003;**95**:1772-1783

[15] Adelstein DJ, Ridge JA, Gillison ML, Chaturvedi AK, D'Souza G, Gravitt PE, et al. Head and neck squamous cell cancer and the human papilloma virus: Summary of a National Cancer Institute State of the Science Meeting. November 9-10, 2008. Washington, DC: Head Neck. Nov 2009;**31**(11):1393-1422

[16] Begum S, Westra WH. Basaloid squamous cell carcinoma of the head and neck is a mixed variant that can be further resolved by HPV status. The American Journal of Surgical Pathology. 2008;**32**:1044-1050

[17] International Agency for Research on Cancer. List of Classifications by cancer sites with sufficient or limited evidence in humans. IARC Monographs on the Identification of Carcinogenic Hazards to Humans. Vols. 1-127. IARC; 2020. Available from: https://monographs.iarc.fr/agents-classified-by-the-iarc/

[18] Freedman ND. Fruit and vegetable intake and head and neck cancer risk in a large United States prospective cohort study. International Journal of Cancer. 2008;**122**:2330-2336

[19] Strati K, Pitot HC, Lambert PF. Identification of biomarkers that distinguish human papillomavirus (HPV)-positive versus HPV-negative head and neck cancers in a mouse model. Proceedings of the National Academy Science USA. 2006;**103**:14152-14157

[20] Fan X, Chen JJ. Role of Cdk1 in DNA damage-induced G1 checkpoint abrogation by the human papillomavirus E7 oncogene. Cell Cycle. 2014;**13**:3249-3259

[21] Hafkamp HC, Mooren JJ, Claessen SM, Klingenberg B, Voogd AC, Bot FJ, et al. P21 Cip1/WAF1 expression is strongly associated with HPV-positive tonsillar carcinoma and a favorable prognosis. Modern Pathology. 2009;**22**:686-698

[22] Preuss SF, Weinell A, Molitor M, Stenner M, Semrau R, Drebber U, et al. Nuclear survivin expression is associated with HPV-independent carcinogenesis and is an indicator of poor prognosis in oropharyngeal cancer. British Journal of Cancer. 2008;**98**:627-632

[23] Faber A. CD44 as a stem cell marker in head and neck squamous cell carcinoma. Oncology Reports. 2011;**26**:321-326

[24] Yu SS, Cirillo N. The molecular markers of cancer stem cells in head and neck tumors. Journal of Cellular Physiology. 2020;**235**:65-73

[25] Zhang Q. A subpopulation of CD133 (+) cancer stem-like cells characterized in human oral squamous cell carcinoma confer resistance to chemotherapy. Cancer Letters. 2010;**289**:151-160

[26] Chien H-T, Cheng S-D, Liao C-T, Wang H-M, Huang S-F. Amplification of the EGFR and CCND1 are coordinated and play important roles in the progression of oral squamous cell carcinomas. Cancers. 2019;**11**(6):760. DOI: 10.3390/cancers11060760

[27] Hayes DN, Van Waes C, Seiwert TY. Genetic landscape of human papillomavirus-associated head and neck cancer and comparison to tobacco-related tumors. Journal of Clinical

Oncology. 2015;**33**(29):3227-3234. DOI: 10.1200/JCO.2015.62.1086

[28] Ma C, Quesnelle KM, Sparano A, Rao S, Park MS, Cohen MA, et al. Characterization CSMD1 in a large set of primary lung, head and neck, breast and skin cancer tissues. Cancer Biology & Therapy. 2009;**8**(10):907-916. DOI: 10.4161/cbt.8.10.8132

[29] Cancer Genome Atlas N Comprehensive genomic characterization of head and neck squamous cell carcinomas. Nature. 2015;**517**(7536):576-582. DOI: 10.1038/nature14129

[30] Spence T, Bruce J, Yip KW, Liu FF. HPV associated head and neck cancer. Cancers (Basel). 2016;**8**(8):75. DOI: 10.3390/cancers8080075

[31] Psyrri A, Rampias T, Vermorken JB. The current and future impact of human papillomavirus on treatment of squamous cell carcinoma of the head and neck. Annals of Oncology. 2014;**25**(11):2101-2115. DOI: 10.1093/annonc/mdu265

[32] Zhou G, Liu Z, Myers JN. TP53 mutations in head and neck squamous cell carcinoma and their impact on disease progression and treatment response. Journal of Cellular Biochemistry. 2016;**117**(12):2682-2692. DOI: 10.1002/jcb.25592

[33] Walter V, Yin X, Wilkerson MD, Cabanski CR, Zhao N, Du Y, et al. Molecular subtypes in head and neck cancer exhibit distinct patterns of chromosomal gain and loss of canonical cancer genes. PLoS One. 2013;**8**(2):e56823. DOI: 10.1371/journal.pone.0056823

[34] Beck TN, Kaczmar J, Handorf E, Nikonova A, Dubyk C, Peri S, et al. Phospho-T356RB1 predicts survival in HPV-negative squamous cell carcinoma of the head and neck. Oncotarget. 2015;**6**(22):18863-18874

[35] Burtness B, Bauman JE, Galloway T. Novel targets in HPV-negative head and neck cancer: Overcoming resistance to EGFR inhibition. The Lancet Oncology. 2013;**14**(8):e302-e309. DOI: 10.1016/S1470-2045(13)70085-8

[36] Karim R, Tummers B, Meyers C, Biryukov JL, Alam S, Backendorf C, et al. Human papillomavirus (HPV) upregulates the cellular deubiquitinase UCHL1 to suppress the keratinocyte's innate immune response. PLoS Pathogens. 2013;**9**(5):e1003384. DOI: 10.1371/journal.ppat.1003384

[37] Wagner S, Wittekindt C, Reuschenbach M, Hennig B, Thevarajah M, Wurdemann N, et al. CD56-positive lymphocyte infiltration in relation to human papillomavirus association and prognostic significance in oropharyngeal squamous cell carcinoma. International Journal of Cancer. 2016;**138**:2263-2273

[38] The Cancer Genome Atlas Network. Comprehensive genomic characterization of head and neck squamous cell carcinomas. Nature. 2015;**517**:576-582

[39] Burns MB, Temiz NA, Harris RS. Evidence for APOBEC3B mutagenesis in multiple human cancers. Nature Genetics. 2013;**45**(9):977-983. DOI: 10.1038/ng.2701

[40] Sewell A, Brown B, Biktasova A, Mills GB, Yiling L, Tyson DR, et al. Reverse-phase protein array profiling of oropharyngeal cancer and significance of PIK3CA mutations in HPV-associated head and neck cancer. Clinical Cancer Research. 2014;**20) (9**:2300-2311. DOI: 10.1158/1078-0432.CCR-13-2585

[41] Haraguchi K, Ohsugi M, Abe Y, Semba K, Akiyama T, Yamamoto T. Ajuba negatively regulates the Wnt signaling pathway by promoting GSK-3beta-mediated phosphorylation of beta-catenin. Oncogene. 2008;**27**(3):274-284. DOI: 10.1038/sj.onc.1210644

[42] Wiest T, Schwarz E, Enders C, et al. Involvement of intact HPV16 E6/E7 gene expression in head and neck cancers with unaltered p53 status and perturbed pRb cell cycle control. Oncogene. 2002;**21**:1510-1517

[43] Nishant A, Mitchell J, Frederickcurtis R, Pickeringchetan B, Changryan J, Licarole F, et al. Exome sequencing of head and neck squamous cell carcinoma reveals inactivating mutations in NOTCH1. Science. 2011;**333**(6046):1154-1157. DOI: 10.1126/science.1206923

[44] Eleni MR, Chung CH, Bishop JA, Howard JD, Sharma R, Li RJ, et al. Cleaved NOTCH1 expression pattern in head and neck squamous cell carcinoma is associated with NOTCH1 mutation, HPV status, and high-risk features. Cancer Preventive Research. 2015;**8**(4):287-295

[45] Gauthaman A, Moorthy A. Prevalence of K-ras Codon 12 mutations in indian patients with head and neck cancer. Indian Journal of Clinical Biochemistry. 2021;**36**(3):370-374. DOI: 10.1007/s12291-020-00882-w

[46] Seiwert TY, Zuo ZX, Keck MK, Khattri A, Pedamallu CS, Stricker T, et al. Integrative and comparative genomic analysis of HPV-positive and HPV-negative head and neck squamous cell carcinomas. Clinical Cancer Research. 2015;**21**(3):632-641

[47] Stransky N, Egloff AM, Tward AD, Kostic AD, Cibulskis K, Sivachenko A, et al. The mutational landscape of head and neck squamous cell carcinoma. Science. 2011;**333**(6046):1157-1160

[48] Lin DC, Meng X, Hazawa M, Nagata Y, Varela AM, Xu L, et al. The genomic landscape of nasopharyngeal carcinoma. Nature Genetics. 2014;**46**(8):866-871

[49] Pickering CR, Zhang JX, Neskey DM, Zhao M, Jasser SA, Wang JP, et al. Squamous cell carcinoma of the oral tongue in young Non-smokers is genomically similar to tumors in older smokers. Clinical Cancer Research. 2014;**20**(14):3842-3848

[50] Pickering CR, Zhang J, Yoo SY, Bengtsson L, Moorthy S, Neskey DM, et al. Integrative genomic characterization of oral squamous cell carcinoma identifies frequent somatic drivers. Cancer Discovery. 2013;**3**(7):770-781

[51] Gaździcka J, Gołąbek K, Strzelczyk JK. Epigenetic modifications in head and neck cancer. Biochemical Genetics. 2020;**58**:213-244. DOI: 10.1007/s10528-019-09941-1

[52] Puttipanyalears C, Subbalekha K, Mutirangura A, Kitkumthorn N. Alu hypomethylation in smoke-exposed epithelia and oral squamous carcinoma. Asian Pacific Journal of Cancer Prevention. 2013;**14**:5495-5501

[53] Foy JP, Pickering CR, Papadimitrakopoulou VA, Jelinek J, Lin SH, William WN Jr, et al. New DNA methylation markers and global DNA hypomethylation are associated with oral cancer development. Philadelphia: Cancer Prevention Research. Nov 2015;**8**(11):1027-1035

[54] Castilho R, Squarize C, Almeida L. Epigenetic modifications and head and neck cancer: Implications for tumor